Color Atlas of Local
and Systemic Signs
of Cardiovascular Disease

To my wife Kathleen and my children Gordon and Marian.

Color Atlas of Local and Systemic Signs of Cardiovascular Disease

BY

Franklin B. Saksena, MD, CM, FACC, FACP, FRCP (C), FAHA

Senior Attending Physician 1973–2005, Currently Voluntary
Attending Physician, Division of Adult Cardiology, John H. Stroger,
Jr. Hospital of Cook County
Assistant Professor of Medicine, Northwestern University & Rush Medical School
Attending Physician, Swedish Covenant Hospital
Attending Physician, St. Mary of Nazareth Hospital, Chicago, IL

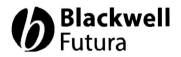

Published by Blackwell Publishing
Blackwell Futura is an imprint of Blackwell Publishing

Blackwell Publishing, Inc., 350 Main Street, Malden, Massachusetts 02148-5020, USA
Blackwell Publishing Ltd, 9600 Garsington Road, Oxford OX4 2DQ, UK
Blackwell Science Asia Pty Ltd, 550 Swanston Street, Carlton, Victoria 3053, Australia

First published 2008

1   2008

ISBN: 978-1-4051-5976-0

Library of Congress Cataloging-in-Publication Data

Saksena, Franklin B.
  Color atlas of local and systemic signs of cardiovascular disease / by Franklin Saksena.
    p. ; cm.
  Includes bibliographical references and index.
  ISBN-13: 978-1-4051-5976-0
  ISBN-10: 1-4051-5976-6
  1. Cardiovascular system–Diseases–Diagnosis–Atlases.   2. Physical diagnosis–Atlases.
I. Title.
  [DNLM: 1. Cardiovascular Diseases–diagnosis–Atlases.   2. Signs and Symptoms–Atlases. WG 17 S158c 2007]
  RC670.S25 2007
  616.1'07500223–dc22

                                                                                    2007017556

A catalogue record for this title is available from the British Library

Commissioning Editor: Gina Almond
Development Editor: Beckie Brand
Editorial Assistant: Victoria Pittman
Production Controller: Debbie Wyer

Set in 9.5/12pt Minion by Aptara Inc., New Delhi, India
Printed and bound in Singapore by C.O.S. Printers Pte Ltd

For further information on Blackwell Publishing, visit our website:
www.blackwellcardiology.com

The publisher's policy is to use permanent paper from mills that operate a sustainable forestry policy, and which has been manufactured from pulp processed using acid-free and elementary chlorine-free practices. Furthermore, the publisher ensures that the text paper and cover board used have met acceptable environmental accreditation standards.

Designations used by companies to distinguish their products are often claimed as trademarks. All brand names and product names used in this book are trade names, service marks, trademarks or registered trademarks of their respective owners. The Publisher is not associated with any product or vendor mentioned in this book.

The contents of this work are intended to further general scientific research, understanding, and discussion only and are not intended and should not be relied upon as recommending or promoting a specific method, diagnosis, or treatment by physicians for any particular patient. The publisher and the author make no representations or warranties with respect to the accuracy or completeness of the contents of this work and specifically disclaim all warranties, including without limitation any implied warranties of fitness for a particular purpose. In view of ongoing research, equipment modifications, changes in governmental regulations, and the constant flow of information relating to the use of medicines, equipment, and devices, the reader is urged to review and evaluate the information provided in the package insert or instructions for each medicine, equipment, or device for, among other things, any changes in the instructions or indication of usage and for added warnings and precautions. Readers should consult with a specialist where appropriate. The fact that an organization or Website is referred to in this work as a citation and/or a potential source of further information does not mean that the author or the publisher endorses the information the organization or Website may provide or recommendations it may make. Further, readers should be aware that Internet Websites listed in this work may have changed or disappeared between when this work was written and when it is read. No warranty may be created or extended by any promotional statements for this work. Neither the publisher nor the author shall be liable for any damages arising herefrom.

Contents

About the author

Franklin B. Saksena, MD, has served as Senior Attending Physician in the Department of Cardiology at Stroger Hospital of Cook County, Chicago, for 32 years. He remains active there as a Voluntary Attending Physician.

While at Cook County Hospital, he was Director of the Cardiac Catheterization Lab and for a period was Acting Chief of Cardiology. In addition, he is an Assistant Professor of Medicine at both Northwestern University Medical School and Rush Medical School. He continues to have a part-time private practice in Cardiology and Internal Medicine at Swedish Covenant and St Mary of Nazareth hospitals.

Educated in England and Canada, he obtained his medical degree at Queen's University, Kingston, Ontario, Canada. He was a Pulmonary Fellow at The University of Chicago for 2 years and spent 3 years as a Cardiology Fellow (Northwestern Medical School and Toronto University hospitals).

He has won a number of awards for excellence in teaching Cardiology and Physical Diagnosis to medical students and residents and continues to be much sought after by medical students and those in the MD, PhD program.

Dr Saksena has written a monograph on *Hemodynamics in Cardiology: Calculations and Interpretations* (Praeger Scientific, New York, 1983). As a Sherlock Holmes enthusiast, he endeavors to apply Holmesian deductions to bedside diagnosis. He is the author of *101 Sherlock Holmes crossword puzzles* (2000). *The Art and Science of Cardiac Physical Diagnosis* by Drs. Ranganathan, Sivacyan, and Saksena, was published in 2006 by Humana Press, Totowa, NJ.

Preface

The early recognition of cardiovascular disease by the Physician is of paramount importance. Cardiovascular disease now ranks as the leading cause of death, resulting in one third of all deaths globally [1] and affecting at least 70 million Americans [2].

A great deal of information about cardiovascular disease can be obtained by the thorough inspection of a patient, using only the unaided senses. However, inspection is a frequently overlooked aspect of physical diagnosis. (We see but do not observe, as Sherlock Holmes was wont to say [3].) Hence, the value of a Cardiovascular Atlas which promotes the recognition of the local and systemic manifestations of cardiovascular disease.

The color photographs are accompanied by explanatory text that describes each physical sign, its utility, and some of its likeliest causes. The rarer syndromes associated with cardiovascular disease are listed in the Appendix.

Whenever possible the physical sign is corroborated with other diagnostic information. I have provided an extensive number of references to acknowledge my debt to other authors and to assist readers should they wish to explore a particular topic further.

I believe that this Atlas will be of use to Cardiologists and Internists as well as those studying for higher examinations.

References

1 Mackay J, Mensah G. *The Atlas of Heart Disease and Stroke.* W.H.O. Myriad Editions Ltd., Brighton, England, 2004. Available at http://www.un.org/Pubs/chronicle/2005/issue1/0105p46.html.

2 American Heart Association. *Heart Disease and Stroke Statistics—2006 Update.* American Heart Association, Dallas, Tx, 2006. Available at http://circ.ahajournals.org/cgi/content/abstract/CIRCULATIONAHA.105.171600v1. Accessed May 1, 2006.

3 Doyle AC. Scandal in Bohemia. In: *The Complete Sherlock Holmes.* Doubleday and Company, Garden City, NY, 1930: 162.

Photographic credits

American Medical Association

Figures 121, 122: Adams SL, Gore M. Diagnostician's digit. A repercussion of percussion. *JAMA* 1997; **277**: 1168. Copyright 1997 American Medical Association. All rights reserved.

Figures 138, 146, 195: Hoeg JM. Familial hypercholesterolemia. What the zebra can teach us about the horse. *JAMA* 1994; **271**: 543–545. Copyright 1994 American Medical Association. All rights reserved.

Figure 186: Secord E, Emre U, Shah BR. Erythema marginatum in acute rheumatic fever. *Am J. Dis Child* 1992; **146**: 637–638. Copyright 1992 American Medical association. All rights reserved.

American Thoracic Society

Figure 109: Waring WW, Wilkinson RW, Wiebe RA *et al.* Quantitation of digital clubbing children. Measurements of casts of the index finger. *Am Rev Respir Dis* 1971; **104**: 166–174.

Annals of Internal Medicine

Figure 14: Daniell HW. Smoker's wrinkles. A study in the epidemiology of "crow's feet". *Ann Intern Med* 1971; **75**: 873–880.

Figure 42: Plotz PH *et al.* Current concepts in the idiopathic inflammatory myopathies: polymyositis, dermatomyositis, and related disorders. *Ann Intern Med* 1989; **111**: 143–157.

Figure 136: Brewer MB, Zech LA, Gregg RE *et al.* Type III hyperlipoproteinemia: diagnosis, molecular defects, pathology and treatment. *Ann Intern Med* 1983; **98**: 623–640.

Figures 137, 196: Leung N, Hegele RA, Lewis GF. Rapid development of massive tendon xanthomas following highly active antiretroviral therapy. *Ann Intern Med* 2002; **137**: 624.

Figures 177, 178: Desnick RJ, Brady R, Barranger J *et al.* Fabry Disease, an under-recognized multisystemic disorder. Expert recommendations for diagnosis, management and enzyme replacement therapy. *Ann Intern Med* 2003; **138**: 338–346.

Blackwell Publishing

Figure 44: Katayama I, Sawada Y, Nishioka K. Facial fold erythema-dermatomyositis. Seborrheic pattern of dermatomyositis. *Brit J Derm* 1999; **140**: 978–979.

Figure 140: Purvis-Smith SG. The Sydney Line: a significant sign in Down's syndrome. *Aust.Paediat J* 1972; **8**: 198–200.

Cardiovascular Medicine

Figure 76: Silverman ME. Visual clues to diagnosis. Williams syndrome. *Cardiovasc.Med* 1985; **10**: 57–61.

Clinical Cardiology

Figures 66, 67: Panossian DH, Marais GE, Marais HJ. Familial endocrine myxolentiginosis *Clin Card* 1995; **18**: 675–678. Reprinted with permission from Clinical Cardiology Publishing Company, Inc., Mahwah. HJ 07430, USA.

Consultant

Figure 34: Lee DV. Myxedema. Photoclinic. *Consultant* 1998; **38**: 300. Copyright 1998 Cliggott Publishing Group. All rights reserved.

Figure 83: Scheiderman H. Macroglossia due to acromegaly. *Consultant* 1992; **32**: 69–70. Copyright 1998 Cliggott Publishing Group. All rights reserved.

Figure 111: Schneiderman H. Digital clubbing due to idiopathic pulmonary fibrosis. *Consultant* 1996; **36**: 1249–1256. Copyright 1996 Cliggott Publishing Group. All rights reserved.

Figure 147: Akritidis NK, Mantzios G, Papaxanthis T. Hemorrhagic necrosis. *Consultant* 1998; **38**: 403. Copyright 1998 Cliggott Publishing Group. All rights reserved.

Figure 167: Zeihen M. Spinal sign for heart disease. *Consultant* 2000; **40**: 1732. Copyright 2000 Cliggott Publishing Group. All rights reserved.

Figure 179: Schneiderman H. Inferior vena cava syndrome. *Consultant* 1991; **31**: 47. Copyright 1991 Cliggott Publishing Group. All rights reserved.

Elsevier

Figures 5, 6, 68, 71: Shapiro LM, Fox KM. *Color atlas of physical signs in cardiovascular disease.* Year Book Medical Publishers 1989. Reprinted with permission from Elsevier. Copyright 1989.

Figures 30, 70, 176: Braverman IM. *Skin signs of systemic disease*, 3rd ed. Saunders, Philadelphia 1998. Reprinted with permission from Elsevier. Copyright 1998.

Figure 31: Bloomfield G, Dunbar K, Wiener CM. Diagnostic dilemma: metabolism. It's all connected. *Am.J. Med* 2006; **119**: 654–656. Reprinted with permission from Elsevier. Copyright 2006.

Figures 32, 41, 95, 96, 148, 185: Forbes CD, Jackson WF. *Color atlas and text of clinical medicine*, 2nd ed. Mosby-Wolfe, London, 1997. Reprinted with permission from Elsevier. Copyright 1997.

Figure 51: Perloff JK. *The clinical recognition of congenital heart disease*, 5th ed. Saunders, Philadelphia, 2003. Reprinted with permission from Elsevier. Copyright 2003.

Figure 79: Zatouroff M. *Physical signs in general medicine*, 2nd ed. Elsevier Ltd, 1996. Reprinted with permission from Elsevier. Copyright 1996.

Figures 84, 93, 94: Mir MA. *Atlas of clinical diagnosis*, Elsevier Ltd, London 1995. Reprinted with permission from Elsevier. Copyright 1995.

Figure 88: Belch JJF, McCollum PT, Stonebridge PA, Walker WF. *Color atlas of peripheral vascular diseases*, 2nd ed. Mosby-Wolfe, 1996: p127. Reprinted with permission from Elsevier. Copyright 1996.

Figure 99: Marks ML, Whisler SL, Clerixuzio C *et al*. A new form of long QT syndrome associated with syndactyly. *J Am Coll Card* 1995; **25**: 59–64. Reprinted with permission from Elsevier. Copyright 1995.

Figure 117: Juergens JL, Spittell JA, Fairbain JF. *Peripheral vascular diseases*, 5th ed, 1980: p557. Reprinted with permission from Mayo Clinic. Copyright 1980.

Figures 54, 199, 200: Perloff JK. The heart in neuromuscular disease. *Curr Prob Card* 1986; **11**: 511–557. Year book Medical Publishers, Chicago. Reprinted with permission from Elsevier. Copyright 1986.

Hodder

Figures 12, 150: Hamilton Bailey. *Demonstration of Physical signs in Clinical Surgery*, 13th ed. John Wright and Sons Ltd, Bristol 1960. Reprinted with permission from Hodder. Copyright 1960.

Humana Press

Figures 7, 8, 20, 33, 35, 39, 40, 48, 52, 72, 85, 86, 97, 104, 105, 106, 141, 164, 166, 169, 187, 189, 190: Ranganathan N, Sivaciyan V., Saksena FB. *The art and science of cardiac physical examination. With heart sounds and pulse wave forms on CD*. Humana Press, Totoya, NJ 2006.

Le Jaq

Figures 25, 26: Bourke K, Patel MR, Prisant LM, Marcus DM. Hypertensive Choroidopathy. *J Clin Hypertension* 2004; **6**: 471–472.

Lippincott, Williams & Wilkins

Figures 56, 57, 58, 59: Taubert K. Diagnostic guidelines for Kawasaki disease. *Circulation* 2001; **103**: 335–336. Reprinted with permission from American Heart Association, Inc. 2001.

Figures 60, 62, 64: Guerrero HG, Campos PM, Harrison CG. Cardiac rhabdomyomas in tuberous sclerosis. *Circulation* 1994; 90:3113–3114.

Figure 100: Bohm M. Holt-Oram syndrome. *Circulation* 1998; **98**: 2636–2637.

Figure 102: Satoda M, Pierpont MEM, Diaz GA *et al.* Char syndrome, an inherited disorder with patent ductus arteriosus, maps to chromosome 6p12–p21. *Circulation* 1999; **99**: 3036–3042.

Massachusets Medical Society

Figures 21, 23, 24: Wong TY, Mitchell P. Current concepts: hypertensive Retinopathy. *New Engl J Med* 2004; **351**: 2310–2317. Copyright 2004. Massachusetts Medical Society. All rights reserved.

Figures 112, 113: Farzaneh-Far. Pseudoclubbing. *New Engl. J Med* 2006; **354**: e14. Copyright 2006. Massachusetts Medical Society. All rights reserved.

Mayo Clinic

Figure 19: Brodland DG, Bartley GB. Kayser Fleischer rings and basal cell carcinoma: fortuitous diagnosis of presymptomatic Wilson's disease. *Mayo Clin Proc* 1992; **67**: 142–143.

Figures 27, 124: Hermans PE. The clinical manifestations of infective endocarditis. *Mayo Clin Proc* 1982; **57**: 15–21.

Figures 77, 78: Blackshear JL, Randle HW. Reversibility of blue-gray cutaneous discoloration from amiodarone. *Mayo Clin Proc* 1991; **66**: 721–726.

Figure 202: Zalla MJ, Su WP, Frasway AF. Dermatologic manifestations of HIV infection. *Mayo Clin Proc* 1992; **67**: 1089–1108.

McGraw Hill

Figures 11 & 98: Rudolph CD, Rudolph AM. *Rudolph's Pediatrics*, 21st ed. McGraw–Hill Medical Publishing Division, NY, 2003. Copyright 2003. All rights reserved.

Radiological Society of North America

Figure 168: Shope TB. Radiation induced skin injuries from fluoroscopy. *Radiographics* 1996; **16**: 1195–1199.

Resident and Staff Physician

Figure 149: Usmani N, Rizvon MK, Mir TP. Heparin induced thrombotic thrombocytopenia syndrome: a clinical review. *Res. Staff Phys* 1998; **44**: 45–52.

Tuberous Sclerosis Alliance

Figures 61, 63: Professional advisory board. Clinical manifestations of tuberous sclerosis. National Tuberous Sclerosis Association, Silver Springs, Maryland.

Authors' permissions

Figure 92: Mount Allison University, Sackville, New Brunswick, Canada. Unknown author, according to Dr Vett, Biology Dept.

Figure 69: Suhonen R. Photo: www.ihotauti.net.

Figure 65: Guerrero, HG (unpublished case).

Figures 22, 29: Solomon M.J.

Acknowledgments

I am indebted to the following Physicians who reviewed sections of the manuscript: N. Ranganathan, Maruti Bhoradi, Mary Klodnycky, Sheridan Meyers, Vahe Sivaciyan. I am responsible for any remaining errors in the book. I would like to thank the physicians at Cook County, St Mary of Nazareth and Swedish Covenant hospitals who referred patients to me.

I appreciate the secretarial skills of Mrs Ruby Stubbs-Stamp who had to frequently retype the many revisions in the text.

Gordon Saksena provided inestimable computer assistance and Marian Saksena provided additional computer assistance and helped in proofreading the text. Librarians, Lizabeth Giese and Olivija Fistovic were most helpful in tracking down references for me. I am also appreciative of Eric Basir's efforts in providing a neutral background for some of the photographs that I had taken. About half the pictures were from the author's collection and the rest were culled from the literature (see photo credit listing page viii). I would also like to thank my wife, Kathleen, who supported and encouraged me throughout the writing of this manuscript.

I am also grateful for the cooperation and encouragement of the staff of Blackwell Publishing, especially, Gina Almond, Beckie Brand, Sally Cowlard, and Namita Sinha.

CHAPTER 1

General observations

Introduction

Cardiovascular examination begins with the inspection of clothed and unclothed patients. The detection of systemic diseases often provides a clue as to the associated cardiovascular problem. General observations include evaluating the weight, the height, the degree of alertness, and the gait. Subsequent observations are organized on a regional approach, starting with the face and ending with the lower extremities. This problem-oriented approach is justified as it mirrors the way a physical examination is carried out. Systemic diseases obviously manifest themselves in more than one region of the body, so some repetition of the clinical findings is inevitable. The examination of the face and hands is especially important in detecting underlying cardiovascular disease. In the legends, the most common cardiovascular entity associated with the depicted sign has been placed in brackets.

Weight

Looking at the patient's own clothing may give a clue to any weight change [1, 2]. Wearing unusually loose clothing may reflect excessive weight loss (Figure 1). The belt may be hitched in several notches (Figure 2) or there may be a loose wedding ring (Figure 3) to indicate weight loss. Cardiac causes of weight loss include advanced heart failure with cachexia or overzealous use of diuretics. Noncardiac causes such as carcinomatosis or anorexia nervosa need to be excluded.

Weight gain may also be assessed by looking at the belt buckle marks to show an expanding abdominal girth as in ascites or obesity (Figure 4). In the latter case, some of the belt marks were obscured by boot polish. Patients with obesity (body mass index over 30 kg/m^2) have a higher incidence of hypertension and diabetes mellitus.

Height

A tall thin person with arm span exceeding the height (Figure 5), a tremulous iris, posterior dislocation of the lens (Figure 6), long thin fingers, a positive wrist, and thumb sign (Figures 7 and 8) [3, 4] are common characteristics of Marfan syndrome [5, 6].[1] In the case (Figures 7 and 8) illustrated, the patient had aortic regurgitation on echocardiography and an enlarged aortic root on CAT scan of the chest (Figures 9 and 10). Aortic dissection is a common complication of Marfan syndrome [5, 6]. A female of short stature (usually <5 feet tall) with webbing of the neck points to Turner syndrome which is associated with coarctation of the aorta in 30% of cases (Figure 11) [7]. A short stature is also seen in William's syndrome (supravalvular aortic stenosis), Ellis–van Creveld syndrome (60% have atrioventricular canal defects), and osteogenesis imperfecta. Patients with osteogenesis imperfecta have blue sclera (Figure 18) and associated aortic insufficiency [8, 9].

Progressive decrease in height and a progressive increase in hat size and saber shin are features of Paget's disease of bone (Figure 12) [10]. Aortic stenosis [11] and left ventricular systolic dysfunction [12] occur in moderately severe Paget's disease of bone, whereas high output failure occurs in patients with more extensive osseous involvement [12].

---

[1]Schwartz (*JAMA* 187:473–479) has claimed that Abraham Lincoln (1809–1865) had Marfan syndrome on the basis of a tall slender appearance, arachnodactyly, hyperopia, and a positive family history. Such skeletal and ocular findings have been challenged by Montgomery (*JAMA* 1964; 189: 165), which in any case are inadequate criteria for making the diagnosis of Marfan syndrome (see Ref. [6]). The history of Marfan syndrome in the Lincoln family is also unconvincing.

Degree of alertness

Patients who frequently fall asleep during an interview may be suffering from sleep apnea syndrome and may or may not be obese (Figures 13) [13]. Sleep apnea is associated with cor pulmonale and systemic hypertension.[2] Other causes of excessive somnolence such as sleep deprivation, boredom, or use of CNS depressants need to be excluded.

---

[2]Sotos JG (*Chest* 2003; 124: 1133–1142) noted that William Howard Taft (1857–1930) probably had obstructive sleep apnea. He was about 6 feet tall and weighed up to 340 lb. He would fall asleep during important diplomatic conversations, while standing up and during meals. These symptoms of hypersomnolence were evident during his presidency (1909–1913). When he had temporarily lost a lot of weight, the President said, "I have lost that tendency to sleepiness which made me think of the fat boy in Pickwick. My color is very much better and my ability to work is greater."

Gait

Muscular dystrophy may present as a high steppage gait [14], whereas Friedriech's ataxia (occurring 1.5/10,000/year) is manifested by a sensory ataxia and pes cavus (Figure 199). Both of these disorders are associated with a cardiomyopathy in over 50% of cases [14]. Tabes dorsalis is characterized by sensory ataxia, optic atrophy, and the Argyll Robertson pupil. There may be coexistent aortic insufficiency due to luetic aortitis [15]. Luetic aortitis is symptomatic in 10% of cases [13]. A festinating gait with orthostatic hypotension is seen not only in Parkinson's disease, but also in the Shy–Drager syndrome [16].

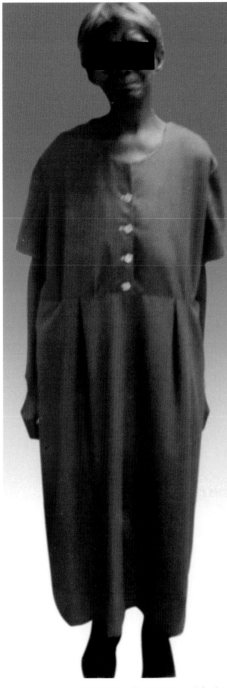

Figure 1 Weight loss: a woman who was treated for heart failure and lost 60 lb. Her clothes now hang loosely.

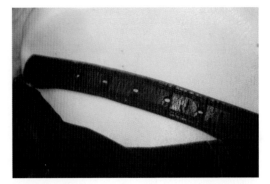

Figure 2 Weight loss: an elderly man who has multiple buckle marks on his belt due to progressive loss of abdominal girth from cardiac cachexia.

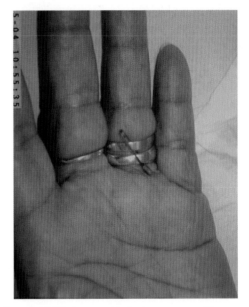

Figure 3 Weight loss: an elderly obese woman with hypertensive heart disease who had lost 40 lb and had to use a safety pin to keep her ring on.

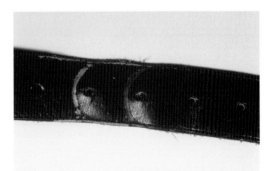

Figure 4 Weight change in obesity: three buckle marks on the belt are seen, one of which has been obscured by black boot polish.

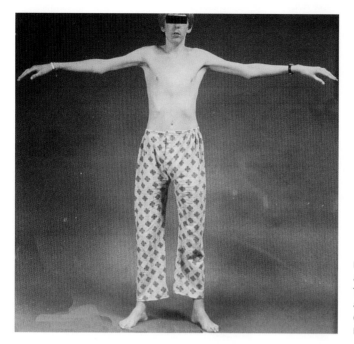

Figure 5 Marfan syndrome: the legs and arms are disproportionately long. The hands may touch the knees and the armspan/height >1 (Aortic dissection). (Reprinted with permission from Elsevier. Copyright 1989)

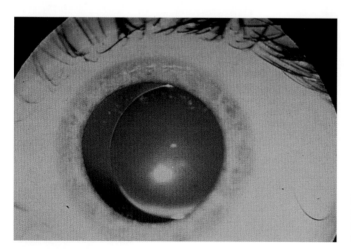

Figure 6 Marfan syndrome: there is posterior dislocation of the lens. (Reprinted with permission from Elsevier. Copyright 1989)

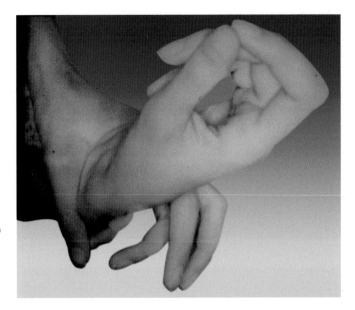

Figure 7 Marfan syndrome: wrist sign in a 24-year-old female. The thumb and fifth finger are encircling the wrist with space to spare. (Reprinted with permission from Humana Press. Copyright 2006)

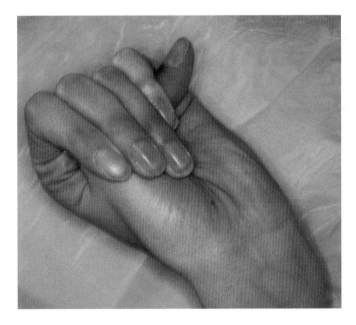

Figure 8 Marfan syndrome. Same patient as in Figure 7, showing the thumb sign in which the thumb can extend across the palm and reach beyond its ulnar surface. (Reprinted with permission from Humana Press. Copyright 2006)

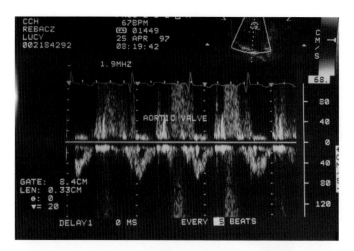
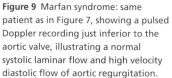

Figure 9 Marfan syndrome: same patient as in Figure 7, showing a pulsed Doppler recording just inferior to the aortic valve, illustrating a normal systolic laminar flow and high velocity diastolic flow of aortic regurgitation.

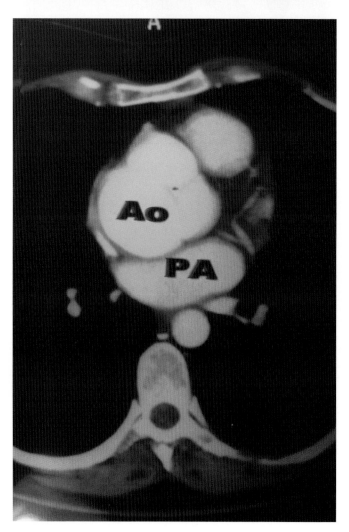

Figure 10 Marfan syndrome: the aortic root of the patient in Figure 7 is dilated to 5.5 cm. The patient subsequently underwent a successful repair of her ascending aorta. Ao, aorta; PA, pulmonary artery.

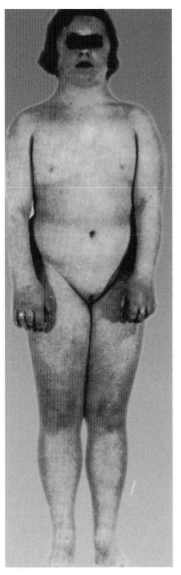

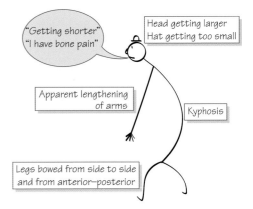

Figure 12 Paget's disease showing in cartoon form its main skeletal characteristics. Modified from Ref. [9]. (Reprinted with permission from Hodder. Copyright 1960)

Figure 11 Turner syndrome: a 15-year-old with a short stature (55 inches tall), webbed neck, increased inter-nipple distance, shield chest, and delayed secondary sexual characteristics (coarctation). (Copyright 2003. McGraw Hill. All rights reserved)

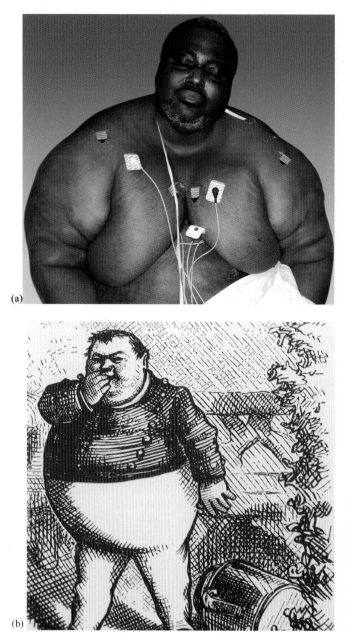

(a)

(b)

Figure 13 Sleep apnea syndrome: (a) this 46-year-old obese man was fast asleep. Height 71 inches, weight 400 lb (cor pulmonale). (b) Thomas Nast's drawing of the fat boy Joe, in the Pickwick papers who was often "in a state of somnolency." (Reference: US edition of Posthumous Papers of the Pickwick Club by Charles Dickens. New York, 1873, as quoted by Burwell CS *et al. Am J Med* 1956; **21**: 811–818.)

CHAPTER 2

Face

Excessive and premature wrinkling (especially "crow's feet" around the eyes) are seen in heavy smokers (Figure 14b) [17, 18] but can also be seen in nonsmokers chronically exposed to sunlight (Figure 14a) [18].

Xanthelasma are multiple, soft, elevated, yellow plaques that usually occur near the inner canthi bilaterally (Figure 15). About 50% of patients will have a lipid abnormality [19]. Pallor of the inferior conjunctival rim points to anemia [20], which may account for a pulmonary flow murmur, a bruit de diable, or high output failure [21]. The latter occurs when the hemoglobin is ≤50% of normal [21]. Dark red conjunctiva in the absence of conjunctivitis may suggest polycythemia (see Figure 16 depicting a 22-year-old man with tetralogy of Fallot; the hemoglobin was 19 g%). Subconjunctival petechiae are seen in systemic infections such as infective endocarditis (IE) [22] (Figure 17). Mild scleral icterus is seen in hepatic congestion caused by right heart failure, pulmonary infarction, chronic constrictive pericarditis, or chronic tricuspid regurgitation. Blue sclerae (Figure 18) are noted in osteogenesis imperfecta, which are associated with aortic or mitral regurgitation [23]. Blue sclera may also be seen in Marfan syndrome [5, 6]. Ehlers–Danlos syndrome [24], Turner syndrome [24], or normal healthy infants <1 year of age as seen in Figure 18.

Arcus cornea is a gray yellow band up to 1.5 mm wide that may encircle the rim of the cornea. It occurs with aging [25] but if seen before the age of 40, it may be a marker of coronary artery disease (CAD) [25]. The presence of a premature arcus (<40 years of age) and xanthelasma may be seen in familial hypercholesterolemia [25]. Arcus cornea is usually bilateral. Unilateral arcus is very rare—it suggests carotid artery stenosis on the non-arcus side [26] provided that ocular hypotony has been excluded [25]. Kayser–

Fleischer rings are diagnostic of Wilson's disease (cardiomyopathy). These rings are brown and encircle the perimeter of the cornea (Figure 19). Hypertelorism (Figure 20) is a feature of LEOPARD syndrome, Noonan's syndrome, pulmonic stenosis with atrial septal defect (ASD), Hurler's syndrome (gargoylism), or supravalvular aortic stenosis [27].

Subluxation of the lens may be seen in Marfan syndrome [5, 6] (Figure 6) or Homocystinuria [28]. Homocystinuria is associated with coronary, cerebral, and renal artery thromboses [29]. Funduscopic findings of diabetes and retinal vessel disease are well described elsewhere [30].

Hypertensive retinopathy is graded according to the Keith–Wagner–Barker Criteria [31].

Grade 1: There is generalized narrowing of the arterioles so that the normal arteriovenous (AV) ratio of 2/3 is reduced to 1/3 or less.

Grade 2: There is further narrowing of the arterioles with sometimes focal areas of spasm. AV nicking is seen.

Grade 3: The arterioles have a reddish brown hue (copper wire). AV nicking becomes more pronounced. Hemorrhages and exudates are now seen.

Grade 4: The arterioles appear like white threads (silver wire). There are pronounced AV nicking, hemorrhages, exudates, and the development of papilledema.

Sequential retinal photography and fluorescein angiography allow a more objective assessment of hypertensive retinopathy than ophthalmoscopy and form the basis for a simplified classification of hypertensive retinopathy [32]:

(a) *Mild retinopathy*: This consists of generalized or localized arteriolar narrowing, AV nicking, and "copper wiring" (Figures 21 and 22).

(b) *Moderately severe retinopathy*: This consists of hemorrhages and/or exudates and microaneurysms (Figure 23).

(c) *Severe retinopathy*: This includes the addition of optic nerve edema to the findings of a moderate retinopathy (Figure 24). Other causes of optic nerve edema such as ischemic optic neuritis need to be excluded.

Patients with a mild retinopathy may be either prehypertensive or have had hypertension for at least 6 years. Preexistent CAD is often seen in such patients [32].

Patients with moderately severe hypertensive retinopathy are strongly associated (odds ratio >2) with stroke and cardiovascular death [32].

Severe hypertensive retinopathy is seen in malignant or accelerated hypertension, which is associated with a further increase in mortality from cerebral or cardiovascular events [32]. Choroidopathy is a less common feature of malignant hypertension, occurring in younger patients whose vessels are pliable and not sclerotic. Choroidopathy may result in retinal detachment and choroidal ischemia (Elschnig spots and Siegrist streaks) [33] (Figures 25 and 26).

Flame-shaped hemorrhages (Figure 27) and Roth spots (Figure 28) are seen in bacterial endocarditis [34], but may also be seen in anemia, leukemia, collagen diseases, or bacteremia [35]. A Hollenhorst plaque is a cholesterol-laden crystal that embolizes to the retinal arteriole usually from an ipsilateral atherosclerotic carotid artery or less often from the aorta or valves [30]. These emboli are white to yellow and refractile (Figure 29). Angioid streaks (Figure 30) and retinal hemorrhages are seen in pseudoxanthoma elasticum (PXE). The retinal vessels and retina appear pale pink in lipemia retinalis (plasma Triglyceride >3000 mg%) (Figure 31). Unilateral prominence of the superficial temporal artery may be seen in ipsilateral internal carotid artery stenosis [36] or temporal arteritis [37] (Figure 32). Patients with internal carotid artery stenosis have an increase in blood flow in the ipsilateral external carotid artery, so that its superficial temporal artery branch is more prominent than on the nonobstructed side (Olivarius's external carotid sign [36]). In temporal arteritis, patients have a tender, ropy, pulseless superficial temporal artery. There may be lingual gangrene, jaw claudication, and later blindness [37].

Endocrine diseases such as myxedema, hyperthyroidism, acromegaly, and Cushing's disease are often detected by looking at the face:

(a) *Myxedema* (Figures 33 and 34): Periorbital puffiness, brittle hair, dry skin, slowing of cerebration, low husky voice, and delayed relaxation of heel reflexes are the main clinical features of Myxedema. The facial features of myxedema are seen in Figure 33. Myxedema is associated with pericardial effusion that rarely leads to cardiac tamponade [38]. Thyroid replacement may lead to a striking improvement in the facies (Figure 34).

(b) *Hyperthyroidism*: Lid lag, exophthalmos (Figure 35), ophthalmoplegia (Figure 36) are readily detected in the established case. Other features such as palmar erythema, fine tremor of outstretched hands, warm moist palms, proximal myopathy, pretibial myxedema, and an enlarged thyroid (Figure 37) are often present. Hyperthyroidism may be associated with high output failure, atrial fibrillation, or a cardiomyopathy [39]. In Figure 38, the patient had hyperthyroidism in the absence of eye signs. He had atrial fibrillation and cardiomyopathy. Temporal muscle wasting was also present.

(c) *Acromegaly*: The lantern jaw, coarsening of facial features (compared to an old photograph), widely spaced teeth, and spade-shaped hands are the usual features of acromegaly [40] (Figures 39 and 40). Acromegaly is associated with hypertension of the low renin type in 18–41% of cases [40]. Coronary atherosclerosis occurs prematurely because hypertension and diabetes frequently coexist in acromegaly. In the example (Figures 39 and 40), the patient had had a myocardial infarct at the age of 40. A specific cardiomyopathy associated with acromegaly remains unproven [40].

(d) *Cushing's disease*: The moon facies (Figure 41), buffalo hump, truncal obesity with thin limbs, and red abdominal striae (Figure 176) are the usual features of Cushing's disease. It is associated with hypertension in 80% of cases [41].

Collagen diseases may also be diagnosed by inspection of the face:

(a) *Dermatomyositis*: A blue-purplish discoloration around the upper eyelids (heliotrope) (Figure 42) along with a raised violaceous scaly eruption over the knuckles (Figure 43) is seen in dermatomyositis [42]. Facial fold erythema has also been described in dermatomyositis [43] (Figure 44). Dermatomyositis can result in congestive heart failure secondary to myocarditis. Pericarditis and heart block rarely occur [44].

(b) *Scleroderma*: The skin over the face may be shiny, smooth, and taut (Figure 45) and it may show mat telangiectasia (Figure 46). The mouth may only be able to open to a limited degree. The dorsum of the hands may also show a taut skin (Figure 47) along with an evidence of Raynaud's phenomenon. Scleroderma is commonly associated with pulmonary hypertension, symptomatic pericarditis in 15% of cases [45], and depressed left ventricular function in <5% of cases [46].

(c) *Disseminated lupus erythematosis (DLE)*: The characteristic malar butterfly skin lesion in the Caucasian consists of a reddish confluent maculopapular eruption with fine scaling involving the nose and cheeks. However, in Black patients with DLE, there is depigmentation in the malar area (Figure 48). Seborrheic dermatitis may also cause a butterfly eruption, which is readily distinguished from that caused by DLE. In seborrheic dermatitis, the eruption extends to other parts of the face and is more scaly [47]. DLE is associated with clinically evident pericarditis in 25% of cases, cardiomyopathy in 10%, symptomatic coronary arteriosclerosis in 10%, and rarely aortic or mitral regurgitation [48–51]. Coronary artery aneurysms may very rarely be seen in DLE [52].

Cardiovascular drugs such as procaine amide, hydralazine, amiodarone, and alpha methyl dopa may produce a lupus-like syndrome, but the butterfly eruption is rarely seen [53]. Pericarditis may occasionally be seen with procaine amide or hydralazine use [54].

Miscellaneous facial findings

Down syndrome (Figures 49 and 50) occurs in 1:1000 newborns and is readily recognized by looking at the face: the vacant unhappy expression, slant of the palpebral fissures, and Brushfield spots (Figure 51). Additional findings include a Simian crease (50% of cases), short stubby fingers (Figure 49), and a small fifth digit [55]. Down syndrome is associated with common atrioventricular canal, ventricular septal defect (Figure 50), and tetralogy of Fallot in 60, 29, and 15% of cases, respectively [56].

A Simian crease may, however, be seen in Noonan's syndrome [57, 58] and sometimes in otherwise normal people [59] (Figure 139).

Patients with the LEOPARD syndrome have *L*entigenes, *E*lectrocardiographic conduction defects, *O*cular-hypertelorism, *P*ulmonary stenosis, and other cardiac abnormalities, *A*bnormalities of genitalia-hypogonadism, *R*etardation of growth, and *D*eafness-sensorineural [60]. Lentigenes (Figure 52) are brown macules up to 5 mm in diameter that appear on the neck, chest, and back. They may increase with age and unlike freckles do not increase with exposure to sunlight. Cardiac abnormalities consist of bundle branch block, pulmonary stenosis, or hypertrophic cardiomyopathy (Figure 53). The latter occurs in 20% of patients with LEOPARD syndrome and as a result such patients may present as cardiac arrest [61].

Patients with Noonan's syndrome [57] have hypertelorism, mental retardation, high-arched palate, webbing of the neck, cryptorchidism, and pulmonary stenosis [58].

Myotonia dystrophica (Figure 54) may produce a masklike face, drooping eyelids, frontal baldness, and sunken cheeks. The His-Purkinje system is involved in 80% of cases and rarely leads to complete heart block [62]. Cardiomyopathy may also rarely occur [62].

The Kearns–Sayre syndrome (Figure 55) consists of bilateral asymmetric ptosis, progressive ophthalmoplegia, and retinal pigmentation. These patients may have complete heart block or rarely a cardiomyopathy [62].

Kawasaki syndrome is usually seen in childhood, mostly in the Japanese. It is an acute febrile disease associated with a widespread vasculitis. There is a nonexudative bulbar conjunctivitis (Figure 56) with relative sparing of the palpebral conjunctiva, the lips are dry, reddened, or fissured, the tongue is strawberry red, and there is pharyngitis. There may be edema and redness of the hands and feet, followed by periungal desquamation of the fingertips (Figure 57), an acute nonsuppurative cervical lymphadenopathy, and a generalized morbilliform eruption (Figure 58) [63]. Kawasaki syndrome is associated with coronary artery aneurysms in 25% of cases (Figure 59), which had a high incidence of occlusion or rupture [64–66] prior to the introduction of high-dose intravenous immune globulin [63, 65].

Tuberous sclerosis is inherited as an autosomal dominant trait (incidence 1:10,000). It is diagnosed by detecting angiofibromata of the lower half of the face (adenoma sebaceum). These lesions consist of small, confluent, and glistening red papules (Figures 60 and 61). There is often a history of seizure disorder, a low IQ, and multiple subungal fibromas (Figures 62 and 63) [67–69]. Tuberous sclerosis is associated with rhabdomyoma of the heart in 66% of cases [70] (Figure 64). Rhabdomyomas of the heart may rarely produce outflow tract obstruction (Figure 65), arrhythmias, and thromboembolic disease [67, 68].

The LAMB syndrome consists of Lentiginous macules [71] of the face ("freckling") (Figure 66), Atrial myxoma (Figure 67), Mucocutaneous myxomas (breast, skin), and Blue nevi [71, 72]. This LAMB or Carney complex is autosomal dominant and constitutes 7% of all cases of myxoma [73]. The genetic locus is on chromosome 17q2 [73].

Patients with progeria show premature aging, especially seen in the face. The skin is thin and tight and lacks wrinkles. Alopecia is present. Patients usually die before the age of 15 of an acute myocardial infarction [74] (Figure 68).

Primary or secondary polycythemia is detected by noting a plethoric or brick red face, dark red conjunctiva (Figures 16 and 103), and a red scalp [75]. Myocardial infarction may occur in primary [76] or secondary polycythemia [77].

Systemic amyloidosis is suggested by the appearance of translucent, waxy yellow papules and plaques on the eyelids, nasolabial folds, and mouth [78, 79]. Purpura frequently occurs in these areas after minor trauma [79] (Figure 69). Restrictive cardiomyopathy is often seen in amyloidosis [78, 80] (see Figure 87).

A violaceous flush associated with facial telangiectasias (Figure 70) or a diffuse erythematous flush (Figure 71) may occur in Carcinoid syndrome in which pulmonary stenosis and tricuspid insufficiency are also seen [81].

The mitral facies consists of venous telangiectasia of the cheeks ("malar flush") and is seen in patients with mitral valvular disease who have a low output state and an elevated pulmonary vascular resistance (Figure 72) [82].

Suffusion of the face may suggest superior vena cava syndrome. The superior cava syndrome may be caused by encroachment of the superior vena cava by an intrathoracic tumor [83], or an aortic aneurysm [84], or thrombosis associated with a transvenous pacemaker [85].

Facial and neck suffusion after elevation of the arms (Pemberton's sign) [86] are seen in patients with subclavian vein thrombosis or a substernal goiter [86, 87] (Figures 73 and 74). Patients with substernal goiters may have hyperthyroidism.

Facial edema may also be seen in those patients with very high venous pressure as in chronic constrictive pericarditis, tricuspid valvular disease, or in children with heart failure.

Angioedema of the face (Figure 75) is characterized by brawny edema and may be caused by a variety of immunological and nonimmunological agents [88].

Patients with supravalvular aortic stenosis (William's syndrome) have an elfin face consisting of large foreheads, upturned nose, a long philtrum, enlarged overhanging upper lip, and puffy cheeks [89, 90] (Figure 76).

Patients on long-term amiodarone (600 mg/day for 2 years) [91] may develop a brown or blue-gray dermal melanosis of the face especially of the areas exposed to the sun (Figure 77). It may take several months for the skin discoloration to resolve after stopping the drug [92, 93] (Figure 78).

Cutaneous lesions of sarcoidosis that involve the face may take two forms: red papules about the eyes, nose and nasolabial folds, and mouth which are pruritic and do not ulcerate [94]; purple plaques that produces a bulbous nose, thickened cheeks, and thickened ears (lupus pernio) (Figure 79). Other features of sarcoidosis include erythema nodosum (Figure 185) and occasionally clubbing [94]. Twenty percent of patients with sarcoidosis have cardiac involvement at autopsy [95, 96]. Clinical manifestations of cardiac sarcoidosis include congestive heart failure, ventricular tachycardia, complete heart block, or cor pulmonale [95, 96].

A seventh nerve palsy may be seen in cerebral embolism especially if there is underlying atrial fibrillation, mitral valve disease, or bacterial endocarditis. A seventh nerve palsy along with a history of a tick bite and meningoencephalitis are suggestive of Lyme disease [97]. In about 10% of late cases of Lyme disease the heart is involved, leading to second- or third-degree heart block or pericarditis [98].

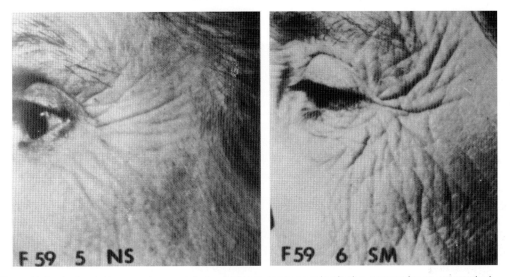

Figure 14 Smoker's wrinkles: excessive crow's feet wrinkling is seen in a smoker (SM) as compared to an age-matched nonsmoker (NS). (Copyright 1971. *Annals of Internal Medicine*. All rights reserved)

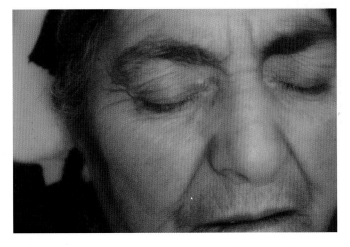

Figure 15 Xanthelasma: the patient had subtle yellow plaques on the eyelids, best seen with the eyes closed (coronary artery disease, hypercholesterolemia).

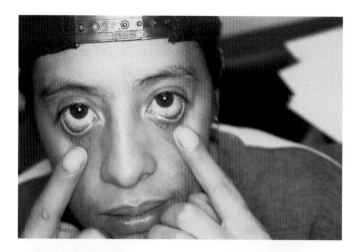

Figure 16 Polycythemia: a 22-year-old man with tetralogy of Fallot. Hemoglobin was elevated to 19 g/dL. He has brick red conjunctiva.

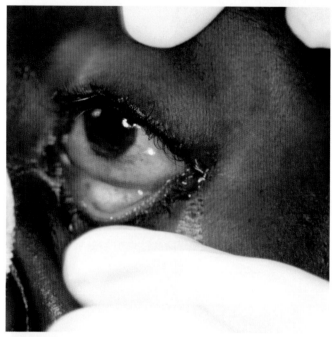

Figure 17 Endocarditis: heroin addict with subconjunctival petechiae and jaundice.

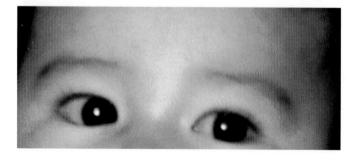

Figure 18 Blue sclera: this is normally seen in infants <1 year old as in this case. Blue sclera in the adult may be seen in osteogenesis imperfecta (aortic regurgitation). In both instances, the sclera is thin and allows the pigmentation of the underlying choroid to show through.

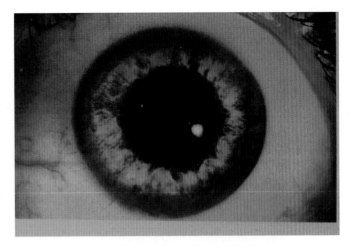

Figure 19 Kayser–Fleischer ring: there is a brown rim of copper deposited around the cornea. The Kayser–Fleischer ring is seen in 95% of cases of Wilson's disease (cardiomyopathy) (Copyright 1992. Mayo Clinic. All rights reserved)

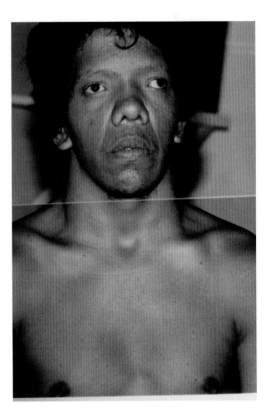

Figure 20 LEOPARD syndrome: this Mexican male has hypertelorism webbing of neck and widely spaced nipples. He also had a Simian crease (cf. Figures 49 and 139), hypertrophic cardiomyopathy (Figure 40), and multiple lentigenes (Figure 41). Strabismus was an incidental finding. (Reprinted with permission from Humana Press. Copyright 2006)

Arteriole

Vein

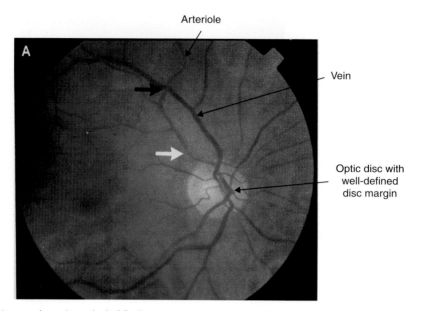

Optic disc with
well-defined
disc margin

Figure 21 Hypertensive retinopathy (mild). There is arteriovenous nicking (black arrow) and focal arteriolar narrowing (white arrow).

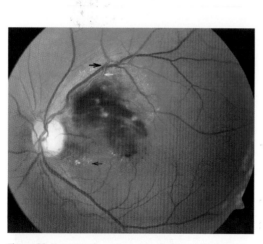

Figure 22 Hypertensive retinopathy (moderate). There is A-V nicking and silver wiring of the superior temporal artery (upper arrow). There is an extensive hemorrhage just temporal to the optic disc as well as "hard exudates" (lower arrow) (Courtesy of Dr. M.J. Solomon, Retina associates)

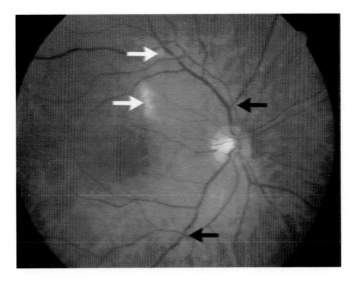

Figure 23 Hypertensive retinopathy (moderate). There is arteriovenous nicking (black arrows) and cotton wool spots (white arrows).

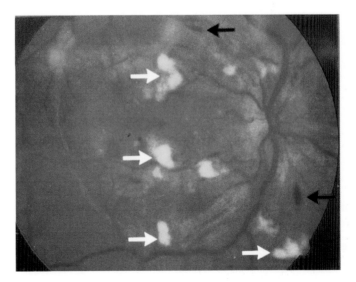

Figure 24 Malignant hypertensive retinopathy. There are several fluffy exudates (white arrows), retinal hemorrhages (black arrows), and papilledema, and there is blurred disc margin.

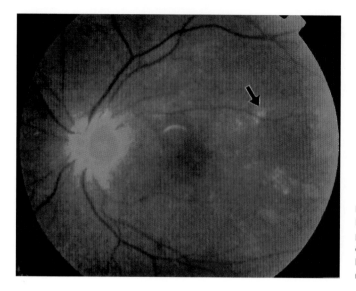

Figure 25 Hypertensive choroidopathy. Elschnig spots (black arrow) are yellow patches of retinal pigment epithelium overlying infarcted choriocapillaris lobules. (Copyright 2004. LE JAQ. All rights reserved)

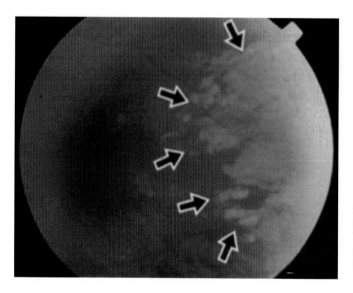

Figure 26 Hypertensive choroidopathy. Siegrist streaks (arrows) are linear hypopigmented areas over choroidal arteries. Later these streaks become hyperpigmented. (Copyright 2004. LE JAQ. All rights reserved)

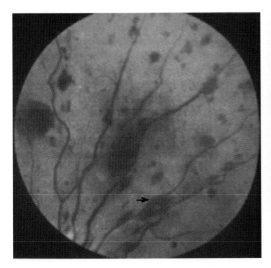

Figure 27 Retinal hemorrhages: this patient had endocarditis. There is a micro-infarct (Roth spot) (arrow). (Copyright 1982. Mayo Clinic. All rights reserved)

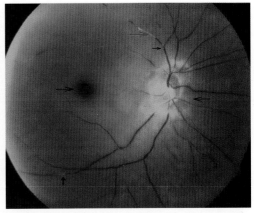

Figure 29 Retinal emboli: Hollenhorst plaques are seen at arterial bifurcations (see black arrows) and represent cholesterol emboli. Extensive fibrinoplatelet emboli are also seen (red arrow) involving most of the superior temporal arteries. The cherry red macula and blurring of the optic disc are signs of the resultant retinal arterial occlusion. (Courtesy of Dr. M.J. Solomon, Retina associates)

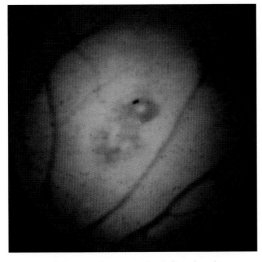

Figure 28 Roth spot: there is a microinfarct (a pale area surrounded by a red zone) in a patient with endocarditis.

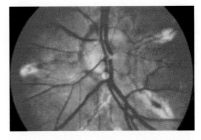

Figure 30 Pseudoxanthoma elasticum: the retina shows angioid streaks radiating from the optic disc in a spoke-like fashion. Angioid streaks are also seen in Paget's disease, Sickle cell disease, Ehlers–Danlos syndrome. (Reprinted with permission from Elsevier. Copyright 1998) (Reference: Kaiser et al. Massachusetts Eye and Ear Infirmary Illustrated Manual of Ophthalmology, 2nd edn., W.B. Saunders, 1994: 333.)

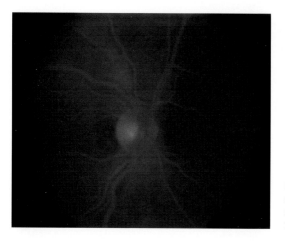

Figure 31 Lipemia retinalis: the retinal vessels are creamy white. Triglyceride level 14,430 mg%. (Reprinted with permission from Elsevier. Copyright 2006)

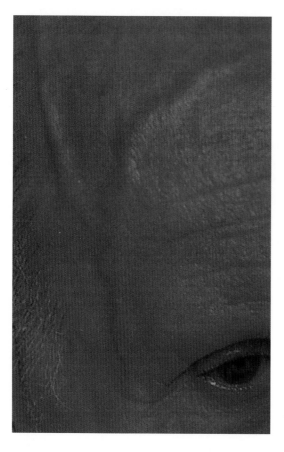

Figure 32 Temporal arteritis: the superficial temporal artery is prominent, thickened, painful, and associated with visual impairment in the right eye. (Reprinted with permission from Elsevier. Copyright 1997)

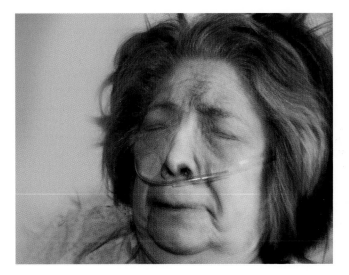

Figure 33 Myxedema: elderly woman who had stopped her thyroid medication for about 1 year. She had coarse hair, dry skin, and a pasty colored face.

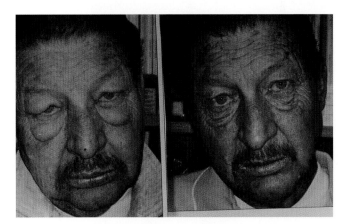

Figure 34 Myxedema: the patient had periorbital puffiness almost closing his eyes, which has disappeared since thyroxine therapy (pericardial effusion). (Copyright 1998. Cliggott Publishing Group. All rights reserved)

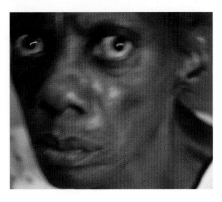

Figure 35 Hyperthyroidism: the patient has visible sclera below the cornea (exophthamos) and sclera visible about the cornea (lid lag). Facial wasting is also seen. (Reprinted with permission from Humana Press. Copyright 2006)

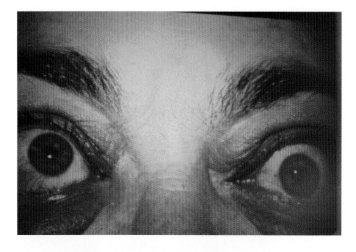

Figure 36 Hyperthyroidism: the patient has exophthalmos and ophthalmoplegia.

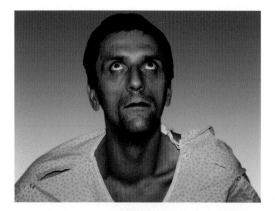

Figure 37 Hyperthyroidism: the thyroid is visibly enlarged in the neck. The I^{131} uptake was increased to 78%.

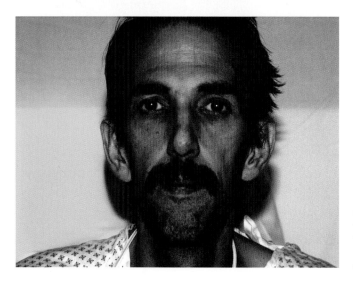

Figure 38 Hyperthyroidism without eye changes: a 40-year-old man who had weight loss, cardiomyopathy, and atrial fibrillation. He responded well to antithyroid medication and subsequently radioiodine (^{131}I).

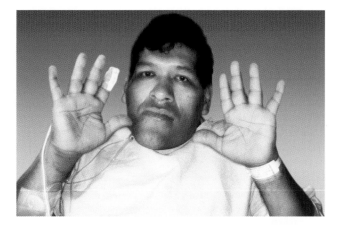

Figure 39 Acromegaly: a 40-year-old man with a lantern jaw, coarse facial features, large spade-like hands. Admitted with an acute inferior wall infarction. (Reprinted with permission from Humana Press. Copyright 2006)

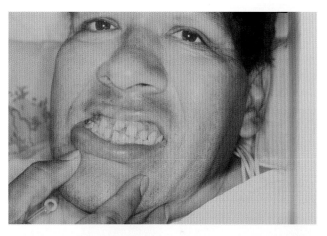

Figure 40 Acromegaly: same 40-year-old man with acromegaly and widely spaced teeth. (Reprinted with permission from Humana Press. Copyright 2006)

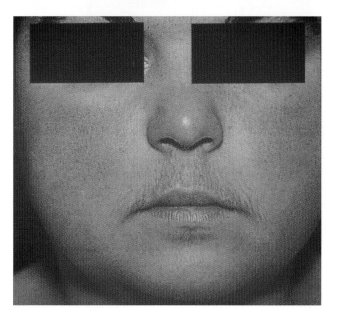

Figure 41 Cushing's disease: this woman has a plethoric moon facies and some hirsutism (hypertension). (Reprinted with permission from Elsevier. Copyright 1997)

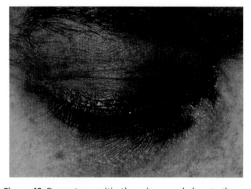

Figure 42 Dermatomyositis: there is a purple hue to the upper eyelids called heliotrope because of its resemblance to a sunflower having reddish-purple petals (myocarditis). (Copyright 1989. *Annals of Internal Medicine*. All rights reserved)

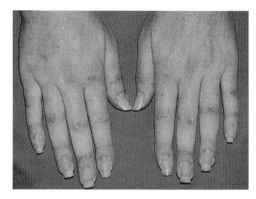

Figure 43 Dermatomyositis: red papules are seen over the inter-phalangeal joints (Gottron's sign).

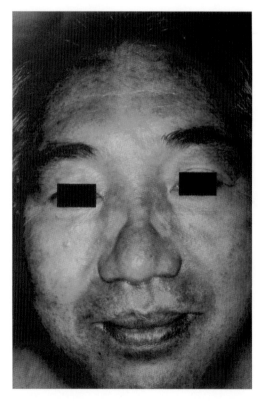

Figure 44 Dermatomyositis: Japanese patient with erythema of the nasolabial and orbital skin folds. (Copyright 1999. Blackwell. All rights reserved).

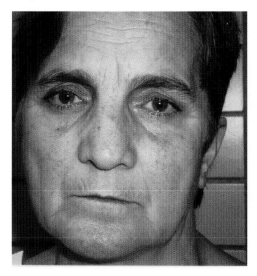

Figure 45 Scleroderma: the face appears masklike with tightening of the skin, radial perioral furrowing, and thinning of lips (pulmonary hypertension).

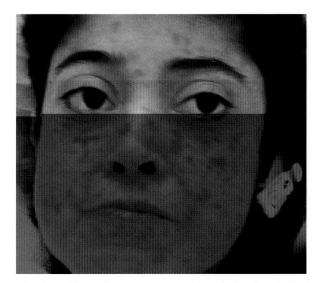

Figure 46 Scleroderma: the face is masklike with mat or rectangular shaped telangiectasia. She had pulmonary hypertension with a mean pulmonary artery pressure of 48 mm Hg.

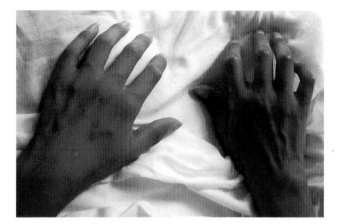

Figure 47 Sclerodema: the skin over the dorsum of the hands and fingers is taut. Same patient as in Figure 45.

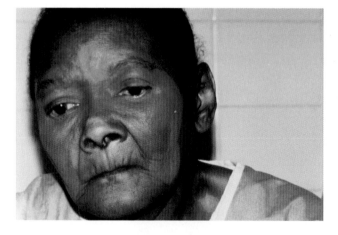

Figure 48 Mixed connective tissue disorder: there is depigmentation of the malar area (corresponding to the malar butterfly eruption seen in Caucasians with disseminated lupus erythematosus). The skin over the face is tight and smooth Radial perioral furrowing is well seen (scleroderma). Rheumatoid arthritis is seen in the hands (Figure 97). (Reprir d with permission from Humana Press. Copyright 2006)

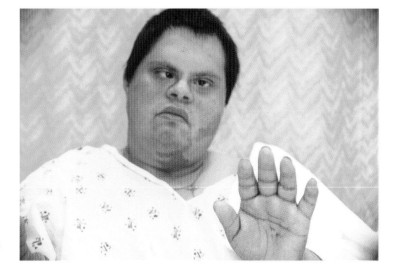

Figure 49 Down syndrome: there is upslanting of the palpebral fissures, epicanthal folds, a vacant and unhappy expression, short stubby fingers, a Simian crease and strabismus incidental finding is a portwine stain on the face.

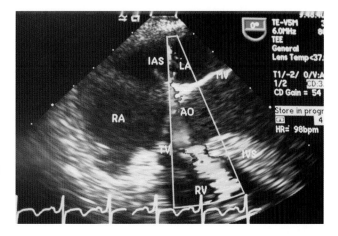

Figure 50 Down syndrome: same patient as in Figure 49. Echocardiogram showing a left-to-right shunt across a small membranous ventricular septal defect using color Doppler flow imaging. Ao, aorta; IAS, interatrial septum; IVS, intervent septum; LA, left atrium; RV, right ventricle; TV, tricuspid valve.

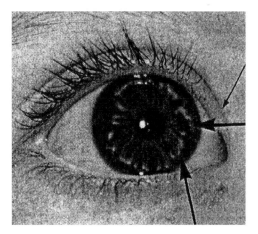

Figure 51 Down syndrome: Brushfield spots are seen in patients with blue irises and consist of white speckles encircling the iris (thick arrows). Thin arrow points to the inner epicanthic fold. (Reprinted with permission from Elsevier. Copyright 2003)

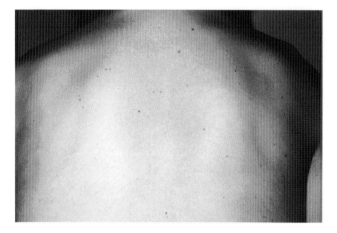

Figure 52 LEOPARD syndrome: lentigenes are seen on the back consisting of l-mm-sized brown macules. Same patient as in Figure 20. (Reprinted with permission from Humana Press. Copyright 2006)

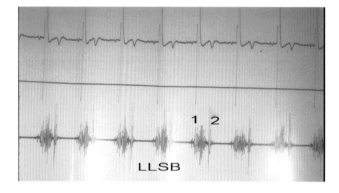

Figure 53 Hypertrophic cardiomyopathy in LEOPARD syndrome. There is a diamond-shaped systolic murmur maximum at the left lower sternal border. Same patient as in Figure 20.

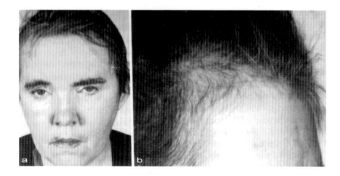

Figure 54 Myotonia dystrophica: (a) this 50-year-old female had an expressionless face, facial weakness, a smooth forehead, and drooping eyelids. (b) A 32-year-old female with frontal baldness and premature graying of hair (heart block). (Reprinted with permission from Elsevier. Copyright 1986)

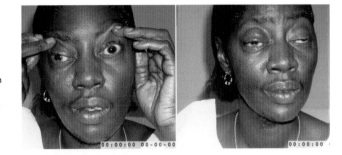

Figure 55 Kearns–Sayre syndrome: a 33-year-old female. On the left, she had an ophthalmoplegia and was unable to move her eyes on request. On the right, bilateral ptosis is seen. She also had retinal pigmentation (heart block, cardiomyopathy).

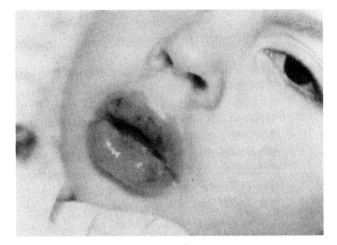

Figure 56 Kawasaki disease: a 2-year-old boy showing conjunctivitis, swollen reddened lips (Copyright 2001. Lippincott, Williams & Wilkins. All rights reserved)

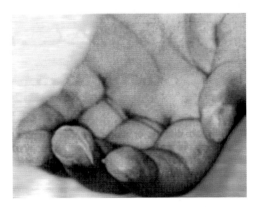

Figure 57 Kawasaki disease: a 3-year-old child with desquamation of the skin around the fingertips. (Copyright 2001. Lippincott, Williams & Wilkins. All rights reserved)

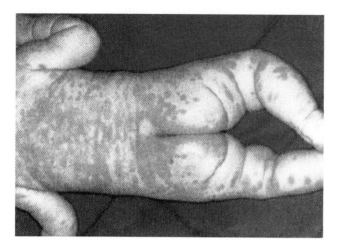

Figure 58 Kawasaki disease: this 7-month-old infant had a morbilliform eruption on her back. (Copyright 2001. Lippincott, Williams & Wilkins. All rights reserved)

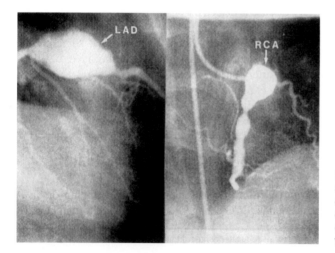

Figure 59 Kawasaki disease: several coronary artery aneurysms are seen in the right coronary artery (RCA) and left anterior descending coronary artery (LAD) in a 6-year-old boy. (Copyright 2001. Lippincott, Williams & Wilkins. All rights reserved)

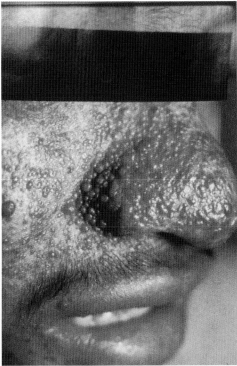

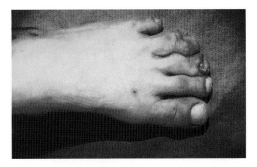

Figure 60 Tuberous sclerosis: a 14-year-old boy with angiofibromata of the lower face.

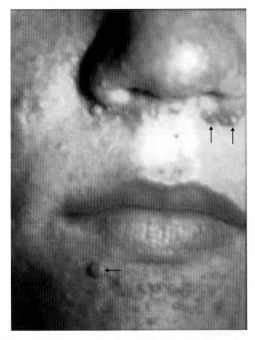

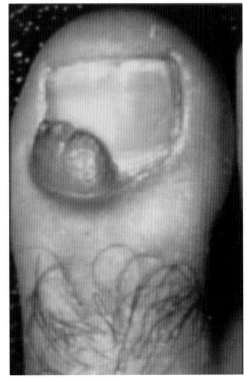

Figure 61 Tuberous sclerosis: early facial angiofibromata (arrows).

Figure 63 Tuberous sclerosis: periungal fibroma of the great toe.

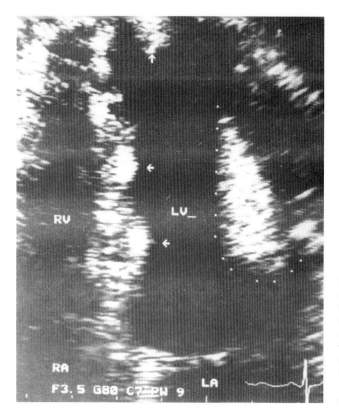

Figure 64 Tuberous sclerosis: same patient as in Figure 60, showing several small tumors involving the apical and septal walls (white arrows) and a 3.5 × l cm mass (partly encompassed by white dots) attached to the lateral wall of the left ventricle on echocardiography in the four-chamber view (probably rhabdomyomas). (Copyright 1994. Lippincott, Williams & Wilkins. All rights reserved)

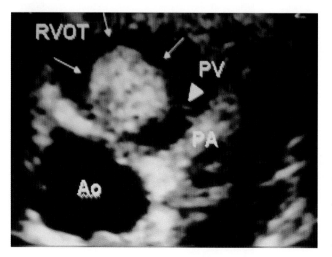

Figure 65 Tuberous sclerosis: a 1-month-old infant with ash leaf skin lesion, pulmonary systolic murmur, and a rhabdomyoma (white arrows) obstructing RV outflow tract. Ao, aorta; PA, pulmonary artery; PV, pulmonary valve; RVOT, right ventricular outflow tract. (H. G. Guerrero, unpublished case)

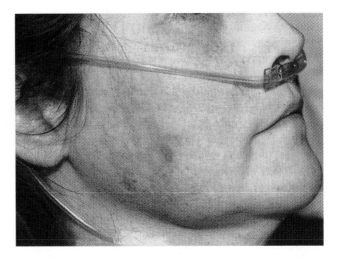

Figure 66 LAMB syndrome: brown red confluent macules are seen over mandibular area and periorbital area. (Copyright 1995. Clinical Cardiology Publishing Company. All rights reserved)

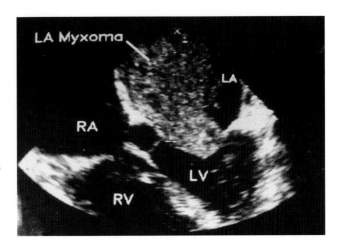

Figure 67 LAMB syndrome. Same patient as in Figure 66, showing a large left atrial Myxoma. LA, left atrium; LV, left ventricle; RA, right atrium. (Copyright 1995. Clinical Cardiology Publishing Company. All rights reserved)

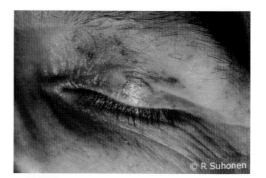

Figure 69 Amyloidosis: hemorrhagic papules on upper eyelids (cardiomyopathy). (R. Suhonen, 2005. Photo: www.ihotauti.net)

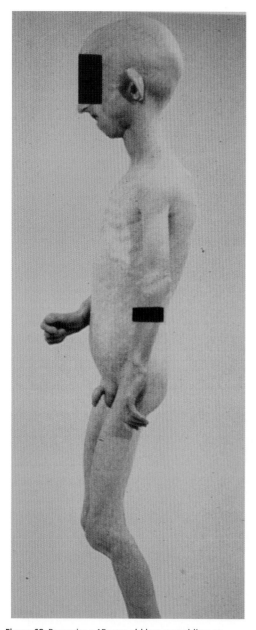

Figure 68 Progeria: a 15-year-old boy resembling an elderly man with a short stature, loss of subcutaneous fat, thin taut skin, and alopecia (premature CAD). (Reprinted with permission from Elsevier. Copyright 1989)

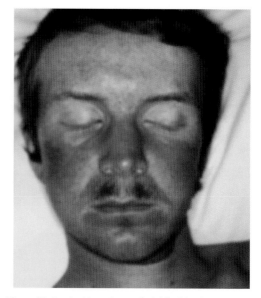

Figure 70 Carcinoid syndrome: facial flushing is seen (tricuspid regurgitation, pulmonary stenosis). (Reprinted with permission from Elsevier. Copyright 1998)

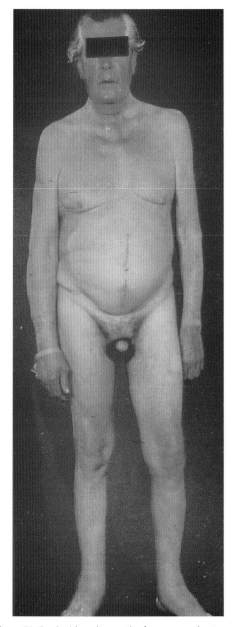

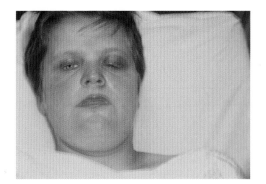

Figure 72 Mitral stenosis: Polish female showing a malar flush. An incidental finding is the false left eye. (Reprinted with permission from Humana Press. Copyright 2006)

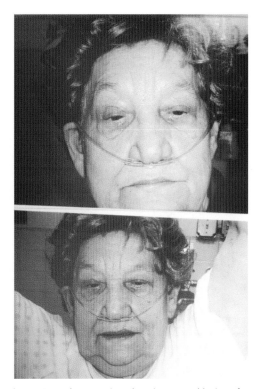

Figure 71 Carcinoid syndrome: the face, upper chest, hands, and knees are flushed. (Reprinted with permission from Elsevier. Copyright 1989)

Figure 73 Pemberton's sign: there is some reddening of the face when the arms are raised overhead (lower picture). She had a substernal thyroid.

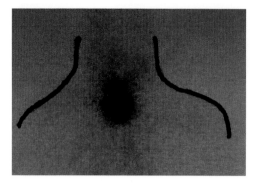

Figure 74 Pemberton's sign: a nuclear scan showing that the patient in Figure 73 had a substernal thyroid. A CT of the chest confirmed that the thyroid extended inferiorly to the great vessels of neck.

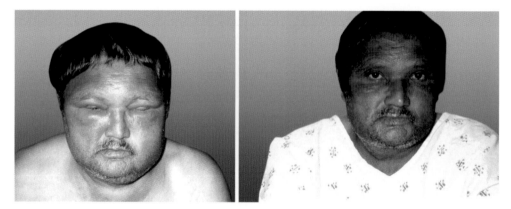

Figure 75 Angioedema of face: the patient had marked swelling of the face of sudden onset. There was brawny edema of the scalp (confirmed by CT of the head). On the right, the patient has improved dramatically in 2 days with steroids. He may have been hypersensitive to enalapril and/or bees.

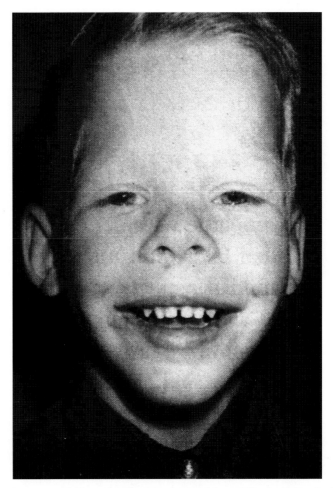

Figure 76 William's syndrome: an amiable youth with a large forehead, long philtrum, overhanging lips, and puffy cheeks (supravalvular aortic stenosis). (Copyright 1985. Cardiovascular Medicine. All rights reserved)

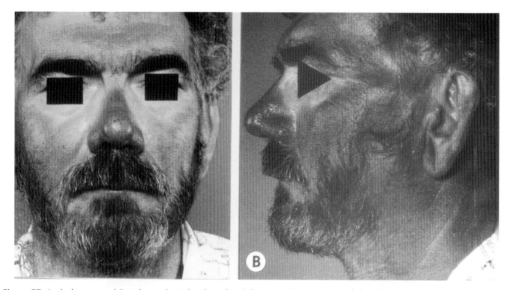

Figure 77 Amiodarone toxicity: the patient developed a violaceous pigmentation of the chin, nose, and cheeks while on amiodarone 600 mg/day for 21 months. An incidental finding is a diagonal ear-crease sign. (Copyright 1991. Mayo Clinic. All rights reserved)

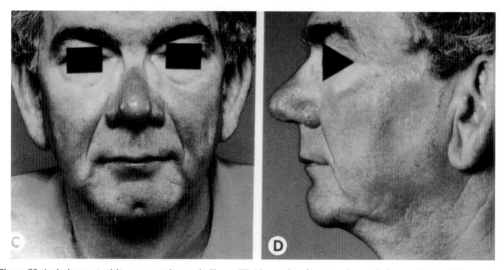

Figure 78 Amiodarone toxicity: same patient as in Figure 77, 18 months after stopping amiodarone. Most of the pigmentary changes have resolved. (Copyright 1991. Mayo Clinic. All rights reserved)

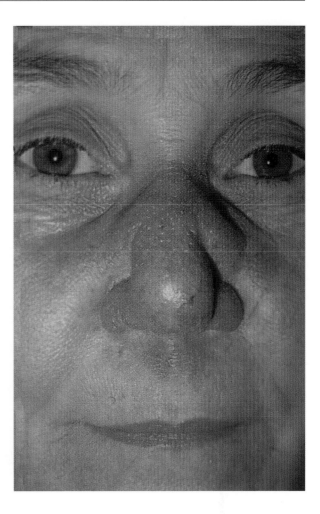

Figure 79 Sarcoidosis: there are pink plaques involving the nose and cheeks (cor pulmonale). (Reprinted with permission from Elsevier. Copyright 1996)

CHAPTER 3

Ear

The diagonal ear-crease sign (Figure 80) [99] is said to be a marker for CAD but the utility of this sign remains controversial [100].[3] If seen in patients <40 years of age, I believe other coronary risk factors should be sought after. Excessive hairiness of the external auditory canal and other parts of the ear in men is also said to be a marker for CAD (Figure 80) but such findings may also be seen in normal subjects [101].

Gouty tophi may be seen on the ear associated with hyperuricemia, which in turn is associated with hypertension. Hyperuricemia occurs in over 25% of patients with untreated essential hypertension [102].

Skin lesions of Sarcoidosis may involve the face and ears (red papulonodules, lupus pernio) (Figure 79).

Congenital deafness may be associated with prolonged QT interval and sudden death (Surdocardiac syndrome) [103]. Thus, the Surdocardiac syndrome should be considered in the differential diagnosis in a child wearing a hearing aid and a history of arrhythmias.

Low slung ears are seen in Noonan's syndrome (pulmonic stenosis), Klippel–Feil syndrome (ventricular septal defect), Turner syndrome (coarctation of aorta), and Trisomy 13 and 18 (VSD) [104]. Small ears are seen in Down syndrome [103].

Generalized darkening of the ears is seen in ochronosis and is associated with aortic or mitral valvular disease [105] (Figure 81).

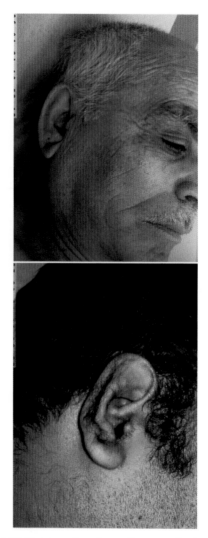

Figure 80 Coronary artery disease. Ear-crease sign in a patient with three-vessel coronary artery disease (upper photo). Hairy ear sign is also seen in coronary artery disease (lower photo).

---

[3]A total of 201 patients (109 male, 92 female) undergoing coronary angiography were evaluated clinically by two observers for the presence or absence of a positive ear crease sign. Mean age $\pm$ 1 SD was 51.1 $\pm$ 9.7 years. The results below showed only a modest sensitivity and specificity for detecting CAD if a positive ear crease sign was present.

	CAD	NO CAD
+VE ear crease	43	22
−VE ear crease	47	89

Sensitivity = 0.66; Specificity = 0.80; Positive predictive value = 0.48 (Unpublished data of Saksena & Enas).

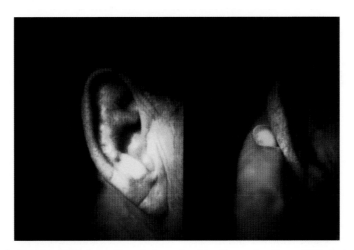

Figure 81 Ochronosis: there is a dark brown-pigmented area involving the ear (aortic or mitral valvular disease). A diagonal ear-crease sign is also seen.

CHAPTER 4

Mouth and nose

Mouth

The tongue may provide a useful clue to underlying heart disease. Central cyanosis is best detected by examining the under surface of the tongue. Common causes of central cyanosis include chronic obstructive lung disease, right-to-left shunts, or polycythemia [106].

The Osler–Weber–Rendu syndrome (Figure 82) [107] is characterized by capillary angiomata of the tongue and lips and is associated with pulmonary AV fistula in 20% of cases [108] or rarely coronary artery ectasia [109]. Other features of this autosomal dominant syndrome are epistaxis and GI bleeding [107].

A chronically enlarged tongue is a feature of acromegaly (Figure 83), hypothyroidism, Down syndrome, or amyloidosis [110]. The patient in Figure 84 had an enlarged misshapen tongue due to amyloidosis. The patient in Figures 85–87 also had amyloidosis with a diffusely enlarged tongue, brown papular eruptions on the back, and a restrictive cardiomyopathy. The myocardium had a sparkling appearance on echocardiography (Figure 87).

An acute swelling of the tongue may be due to bleeding (Figure 88) from anticoagulant use or from angioedema. Angioedema of the tongue is rarely seen after ACE inhibitor drug use (1:3000 patients/week) [110–113]. However, Kostis *et al.* [114] noted a higher percentage of patients developed angioedema associated with enalapril (0.68%) in their prospective series of over 12,000 patients. They noted that angioedema usually occurred in black patients over the age of 65 and within the first month of starting enalapril (Figure 89) [114].

Gum hyperplasia (Figure 90) is seen in patients on Dilantin, cyclosporine, or nifedipine [115]. Steele

et al. noted gum hyperplasia in 38% of patients who had been on nifedipine for at least 3 months [116]. Such patients who develop gum hyperplasia often have poor dental hygiene.

Smoking crack cocaine can lead to palatal perforations or ulcerations due to the high temperature of the inhaled smoke [117, 118]. The user of cocaine may test its purity by rubbing it on the gums to detect its local anesthetic effect. As a result of this practice, gingivitis and enamel erosions on the buccal surface may occur owing to the fact that cocaine is highly acidic [119–121] (Figure 91). Cocaine use is associated with myocardial ischemia or necrosis as well as systemic hypertension [122, 123]. On the other hand, loss of dental enamel (on the lingual surface of the tooth) may occur in bulimic patients who engage in self-induced vomiting in which gastric acid destroys the enamel [124]. Poor dental hygiene in a patient with suspected bacterial endocarditis may suggest a source of the infection. A high-arched palate is usually seen in normals as a genetic trait [125]. It is rarely seen in Turner syndrome (coarctation of aorta) [103], Noonan's syndrome [57], and Marfan syndrome (aortic dissection) [6]. A high-arched palate is only a minor diagnostic criterion for Marfan syndrome [6].

Petechiae on the palate may be due to septicemia such as IE [34]. The deposition of cholesterol esters in the tonsils giving them a bright orange lobulated appearance is seen in familial HDL deficiency (Tangier disease) (Figure 92) [126]. The serum cholesterol is usually below 120 mg%. Other features include premature CAD [127, 128] and peripheral neuropathy [129].

Nose

A saddle-shaped nose is a rare occurrence now. It is associated with syphilis (aortic insufficiency).

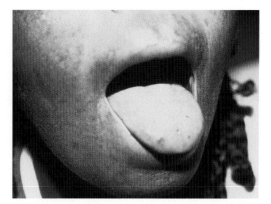

Figure 82 Osler–Weber–Rendu syndrome: there are capillary angiomata on the tongue. She also had telangiectasia of the face and upper chest. (Pulmonary AV fistula).

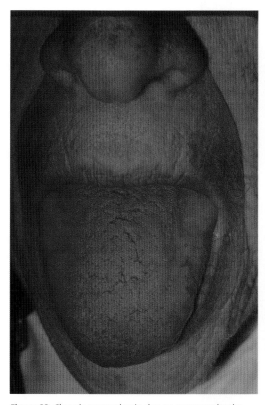

Figure 83 Chronic macroglossia due to acromegaly: the tongue completely filled the opened mouth. (Copyright 1992. Cliggott Publishing Group. All rights reserved)

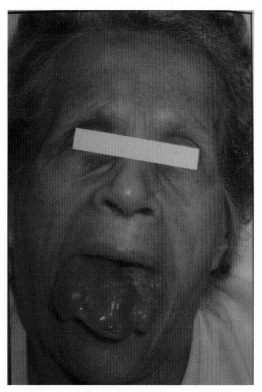

Figure 84 Chronic macroglossia due to amyloidosis: the tongue is irregularly thickened and has a trifid appearance. (Reprinted with permission from Elsevier. Copyright 1995)

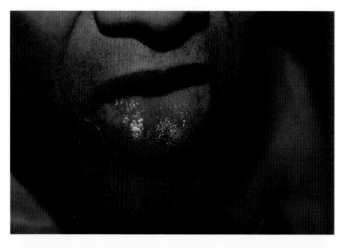

Figure 85 Chronic macroglossia due to amyloidosis: the tongue is diffusely enlarged. (Reprinted with permission from Humana Press. Copyright 2006)

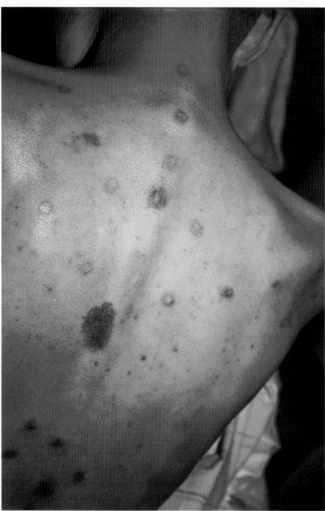

Figure 86 Brown papules are seen over the back. Same patient as in Figure 85. (Reprinted with permission from Humana Press. Copyright 2006)

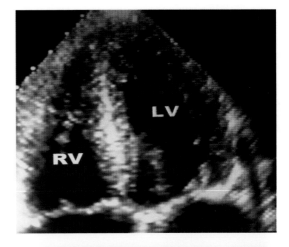

Figure 87 Echocardiogram in apical four-chamber view of patient seen in Figure 85: the myocardium has a glittering appearance and is markedly thickened. The patient was in heart failure due to a restrictive cardiomyopathy. LV, left ventricle; RV, right ventricle.

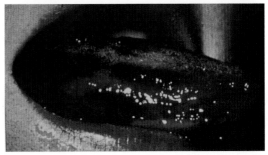

Figure 88 Acute macroglossia: the tongue is diffusely enlarged and bright red along its lateral portion. The patient had bleeding into the tongue while on anticoagulants. (Reprinted with permission from Elsevier. Copyright 1996)

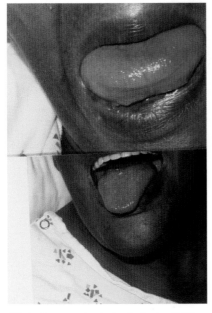

Figure 89 Acute macroglossia due to Enalapril: this 75-year-old Black female developed acute swelling of tongue and lips after being on enalapril for 2 days. She was unable to talk or swallow (upper photo). In lower photo, 2 days after stopping enalapril, the tongue and lips have returned to their normal size.

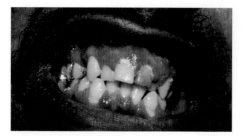

Figure 90 Gum hyperplasia due to Dilantin. Similar findings may be seen in patients on nifedipine.

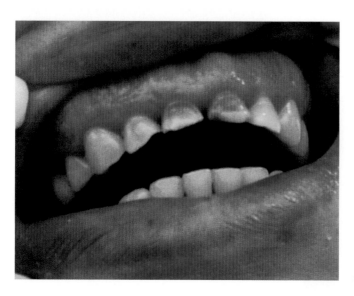

Figure 91 Enamel erosions, best seen on upper incisors and gingivitis due to cocaine (Coronary artery spasm/occlusion).

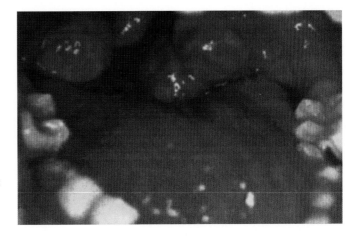

Figure 92 Tangier disease of the tonsils: the tonsils are enlarged with bright orange yellow streaks ("tiger stripes") (premature CAD).

CHAPTER 5

Neck

Inspection of the neck will provide information on the jugular venous pulse and pressure, the thyroid, the presence or absence of surgical scars, an inspiratory tracheal tug sign, webbing of the neck, or PXE.

The technique of examination of the jugular venous pulse requires a combination of inspection and palpation and/or auscultation to properly time the waveforms [130].

Jugular pulsations, in general, are characterized by faster downward movements, namely the X_1 and the Y descents during systole and diastole, being associated with rapid inflow of blood into the right atrium. The slow rates of rise of pressures of A and V waves are not easily seen in the normals. When the rate of rise of the A and/or the V waves are exaggerated and rapid, they can be easily recognized by timing the descents that follow them. The A wave is usually followed by the X_1 descent in normal sinus rhythm which can be timed to systole as judged by simultaneous palpation of the radial arterial pulse. The V wave, on the other hand, is followed by the Y descent, which can be shown to be diastolic in timing. In addition, the A wave and the V wave can also be distinguished by the fact that the A wave rises rapidly and has a shorter duration. The V wave, on the other hand, has a longer duration. Thus, the V wave while it will rise with the arterial pulse and will last longer than the arterial pulse.

The jugular venous pulse may show a prominent A wave due to tricuspid stenosis, pulmonic stenosis, or pulmonary hypertension. The A wave is absent in atrial fibrillation. Intermittent cannon A waves are seen in atrioventricular dissociation. A dominant V wave is present in tricuspid regurgitation or in an uncomplicated secundum ASD. Rapid X_1 and Y descents are seen in chronic constrictive pericarditis. A slow Y descent is a feature of tricuspid stenosis.

A shallow or absent Y descent is a feature of cardiac tamponade [130].

Bilateral neck vein distention may be seen in right heart failure or superior vena cava syndrome. Unilateral neck vein distention may be due to the superior vena cava syndrome. Distention of the left jugular vein could also be due to a kinked innominate vein. In this syndrome, a rigid and probably ectatic aorta presses on the innominate vein to produce a rise in left-sided jugular venous pressure [131]. The thyroid may be visibly enlarged to suggest thyroid dysfunction. A carotid endarterectomy or tracheostomy scar also needs to be noted (Figure 157).

An inspiratory tracheal tug sign is often visible and consists of inferior motion of the thyroid cartilage on inspiration, often associated with tachypnea [132]. It is due to an increased work of breathing and may be seen in congestive heart failure or such pulmonary causes as chronic obstructive lung disease or severe pneumonia. This sign is not to be confused with the tracheal tug in systole due to an aortic aneurysm.

Webbing of the neck is seen in (a) genetic disorders: Turner syndrome (Figure 11) [133], Down syndrome, or Noonan's syndrome (Figure 20); (b) congenital heart disease: hypoplastic left ventricle and secundum ASD [134]; and (c) chromosomal abnormalities [135–139].

Pseudoxanthoma elasticum in the neck consists of a network of closely grouped yellow papules (plucked chicken skin appearance) (Figure 93). The skin is lax and hangs in folds. Similar findings are seen in the axillae (Figure 94), abdomen, and thighs [140]. Angioid streaks and retinal hemorrhages are found in the eyes (Figure 30). It is associated with mitral valve prolapse, hypertension, peripheral vascular disease, and premature CAD [141]. The latter being a common cause of early death [141].

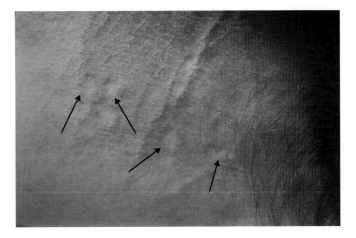

Figure 93 Pseudoxanthoma elasticum: yellow papules (arrows) are present over the entire neck (mitral valve prolapse, CAD). (Reprinted with permission from Elsevier. Copyright 1995)

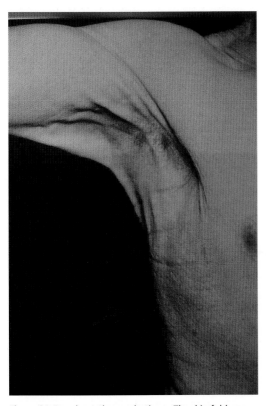

Figure 94 Pseudoxanthoma elasticum. The skin folds over the axilla are lax. (Reprinted with permission from Elsevier. Copyright 1995)

CHAPTER 6

Hand

Examination of the hands provides a most useful mirror of systemic disease [142]. Attention is paid to the size and shape of the hand as well as to the presence of edema, neuromuscular disease, color changes, nail abnormalities, palmar abnormalities, and to temperature changes.

(a) *Size and shape*: Large blunt or spade hands are seen in acromegaly which is associated with hypertension or premature CAD (Figure 39) [40]. Arachnodactyly is seen in Marfan syndrome (Figures 7 and 8) [5]. Hyperextensible joints may be seen in normals, Marfan syndrome [5], PXE [140], and Ehlers–Danlos syndrome (Figure 95). In the Ehlers–Danlos[4] syndrome the skin is also hyperextensible (Figure 96); the cardiovascular associations are aortic dissection, spontaneous aortic rupture, and mitral valve prolapse [142]. Spindle form joints are a feature of early rheumatoid arthritis or DLE, both of which may be associated with pericarditis [142]. Chronic rheumatoid arthritis occurs mainly in women and is characterized by marked ulnar deviation of the metacarpal–phalangeal joints (Figure 97). These patients develop premature atherosclerosis [143]. There is a threefold increase in incidence of CAD if the patient has had rheumatoid arthritis >10 years [144]. Gouty arthritis usually affects a single joint in the hand and may predict a higher incidence of hypertension due to its association with hyperuricemia [102]. Hyperuricemia is also seen in cyanotic heart disease but rarely produces gouty arthritis [145].

The square dry hand is a feature of cretinism (pericardial effusion, pericardial tamponade). A short incurved fifth digit is seen in Down syndrome (Figure 49) [55, 146] whereas short fourth digits occur in Turner syndrome [7] (Figure 98). Syndactyly ("finger webbing") (Figure 99) usually occurs between the third and fourth fingers and while it may be seen in normal subjects, it may also be associated with the prolonged QT syndrome and sudden death [147].

The Holt–Oram syndrome consists of an extra phalanx in the thumb (fingerized thumb) (Figure 100), or absence of the thumb and is associated with a secundum ASD [148–151].

An extra digit (Figure 101) is seen in secundum ASD, Ellis–van Crevard syndrome [103], and Laurence–Moon–Biedl syndrome [103]. A radially curved fifth finger is seen in Hurler's syndrome (multivalvular involvement, cardiomyopathy, CAD) [103]. Absence of the fifth middle phalanges, hypoplastic proximal, and distal fifth phalanges are seen in the Char syndrome (persistent ductus arteriosus, facial dysmorphism) [152] (Figure 102).

Clubbing of the fingers is usually associated with pulmonary disease (80% of cases) [153] with cardiac disease accounting for 10–15% of cases. Cardiovascular associations include right-to-left shunts (tetralogy of Fallot, transposition of great vessels). The patient in Figures 103 and 104 had tetralogy of Fallot with cyanosis and clubbing. Other cardiac causes of clubbing include bacterial endocarditis [153, 154], myxoma of left atrium [155], and rarely an infected abdominal aortic graft [156].

Unilateral clubbing is seen in aortic or subclavian aneurysm or rarely persistent ductus arteriosus with right-to-left shunting and an absent aortic arch [157].

Differential clubbing, in which clubbing is more prominent in the feet than the hands,

---

[4]It was speculated that the inordinate skill of the famous violinist Nicolo Paganini was due to his having the Ehlers Danlos syndrome, which accounted for his hyperextensible fingers and excessive joint laxity. (Smith & Worthington as quoted by L. Jacierno in History of Cardiology, Parthenon, London, 1994, p. 409).

occurs in persistent ductus arteriosus when there is a right-to-left shunt or an infected abdominal aortic graft [156].

The normal angle that the nail plate makes with the adjacent skin fold is 150–170° [158–160]. In clubbing, the nail-bed angle or profile angle exceeds 180° and the hyponychial angle [160] (normal = 178–192°) is increased (Figures 105 and 106).

Normally, there is a window formed between the thumbnails when they are held together and seen in profile (Figure 107). In clubbing the hyponychial angle is increased and the window between the two pressed together thumbnails is lost (Shamroth's clubbing sign) (Figures 108) [161].

A useful sign of early clubbing is to determine if the ratio of the distal phalangeal depth to the interphalangeal joint depth in the index finger exceeds 1.0 (normal ratio using a micrometer is 0.90 ± 0.04) [159] (Figure 109). This distal/interphalangeal ratio may also be visually assessed at the bedside with a "shadowgram" [156].

Subcuticular edema (Figure 110) and ballotability of the nail itself are often present but the latter may be a late sign of clubbing [162]. Clubbing needs to be distinguished from nail beaking and acro-osteolysis. In nail beaking, the nail is curved, the hyponychial angle is preserved, and there is loss of pulp tissue (Figure 111) [163, 164]. Nail beaking is not associated with cardiac disease. Patients with acro-osteolysis exhibit a somewhat flattened and bulbous shape of the distal digits due to soft tissue collapse as a result of necrosis of the distal phalanges. The nail-bed angle is however normal [156, 165] (Figures 112 and 113).

(b) *Edema*: Edema of the hand may be seen in superior vena cava syndrome (Figure 153). Raynaud's disease or thoracic outlet syndrome in which venous obstruction of the upper extremity is present [142] (Figures 114 and 115), but trauma and infection may also produce hand edema [166].

(c) *Neuromuscular disease*: The shoulder hand syndrome is rarely seen in myocardial infarction nowadays, since prolonged immobilization for an acute myocardial infarction is no longer carried out. The hand is swollen and the shoulder is painful to abduct probably from an adhesive capsulitis of the shoulder joint [167].

Thenar and hypothenar wasting may be seen with myotonia dystrophica. The latter is associated with a cardiomyopathy [62].

Fine tremor of the outstretched hands suggests hyperthyroidism.

(d) *Color changes*: Tobacco tar staining of the hands is suggestive of a heavy smoker. The clothing of a smoker may smell of tobacco and show burn marks. Heavy smokers have a higher incidence of CAD, peripheral vascular disease, lung cancer, and emphysema.

Cyanosis of the nail beds is seen in heart failure, Raynaud's disease, polycythemia, obliterative vascular disease, collagen diseases, right-to-left shunts (Figure 103), and cor pulmonale [168].

Cyanosis and clubbing are more prominent in the lower extremities than in the fingernails if there is a persistent ductus arteriosus with a right-to-left shunt or a persistent ductus arteriosus with an aberrant right subclavian artery [106, 169].

Intermittent pallor of the fingers (especially of the second and third fingers) is seen in patients (usually women) exposed to cold with Raynaud's phenomenon (Figures 116 and 117). Raynaud's phenomenon is commonly associated with collagen vascular disease (especially scleroderma) or obliterative vascular disease. Pallor is followed by cyanosis and then reactive hyperemia (Figure 118) [170]. Raynaud's phenomenon is readily distinguished from acrocyanosis as only in the latter is there persistent cyanosis of the fingertips (Figures 119 and 120 depict the same patient) [171].

Diagnostician's digit consists of a rounded red discoloration of the dorsal aspect of the middle finger resulting from using the middle finger as a pleximeter when the heart border is being percussed out (Figures 121 and 122) [172].

Vitiligo is commonly seen in hyperthyroidism (Figure 123) but may also be seen in Addison's disease, pernicious anemia, or in normal subjects [173].

Osler's nodes (Figure 124) are features of septic emboli secondary to endocarditis

[22] or prolonged radial artery cannulation [174]. Osler's nodes are typically painful red subcutaneous nodules 2 mm in size, on the tips of the fingers, thenar or hypothenar areas that disappear after a few days [174]. Janeway lesions are painless red macules or nodules found on the palms or soles [175] and are also a feature of septic emboli secondary to endocarditis. Figures 125 and 126 depict a heroin user with bacterial endocarditis involving the mitral valve producing mitral regurgitation. She had nail-bed hemorrhages (Figure 127) and Janeway lesions on the soles of her feet (Figure 128).

Gangrenous changes in the fingers are seen in Buerger's disease [176], frostbite (Figure 129–131), thoracic outlet syndrome, or vasculitis of any cause. Of the causes of vasculitis, scleroderma is often associated with small areas of necrosis and ulcerations of the fingertips ("rat bite" necroses) [177].

(e) *Nail abnormalities*: Subungal hemorrhages ("splinter hemorrhages") (Figure 127) may be seen in endocarditis and usually involve the middle portion of the nail. They are also seen in scurvy, Osler–Weber–Rendu syndrome or systemic embolism [178].

White nails (Terry's nails) [179] are seen in chronic hepatic congestion (due to heart failure) or low serum albumin (Figure 132, see also Figure 143).

A red lunula is associated with heart failure (Figure 133) [180], but has also been noted in psoriasis and collagen diseases [181]. Blue gray nails are seen in hemochromatosis (cardiomyopathy), Wilson's disease (cardiomyopathy), and ochronosis (aortic or mitral valvular disease) [182]. Black nails are seen in Cushing's syndrome [183] (hypertension).

Onycholysis (Plummer's nails) (Figure 134—same patient as in Figure 35) may be a sign of hyperthyroidism especially if it involves the fourth finger [184]. As there are numerous other causes of onycholysis (such as trauma, chemical trauma, psoriasis, syphilis) [142, 184], onycholysis lacks specificity for hyperthyroidism.

Subungal and periungal fibromas (hands, feet) are a feature of tuberous sclerosis [67] (Figures 62 and 63) (cardiac tumors) (Figures 64 and 65).

(f) *Palmar changes*: Palmar erythema may be seen in normal subjects, hyperestrinism, hyperthyroidism, or beri-beri [185]. Acupuncture palmar marks in a patient on anticoagulants can simulate the embolic phenomenon of IE (Figure 135). Yellowish palmar creases are seen in type-3 broad beta hyperlipidemia (Figure 136) [186].

Xanthomas involving the dorsum of the hand are seen in hypercholesterolemia (Figures 137 and 138). A simian crease is a fusion of the proximal and distal transverse creases of the hand into a single transverse crease. It occurs in 40–50% of patients with Down syndrome [59], and in 5–7% of normal subjects [59] (Figure 139) and rarely in Trisomy 13 [103]. An elongated proximal transverse crease (Sidney line) may also be seen in Down syndrome [59] (Figure 140).

(g) *Temperature change*: Warm moist hands are seen in hyperthyroidism or Paget's disease of the bone—both diseases may lead to high output failure.

Cool hands are seen in hypothyroidism, arterial occlusion, collagen vascular disease, or Raynaud's disease.

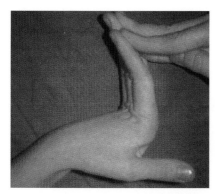

Figure 95 Ehlers–Danlos syndrome (Forbes). The patient exhibits hyperextensible fingers. In some patients, the fingers are able to bend backwards parallel to the forearm on extension of the wrist and metacarpal joints, other criteria* for excessive joint laxity are: (a) elbows and knees extend beyond 180°; (b) the thumb can touch the forearm on flexing the wrist; (c) the foot can be dorsiflexed to 45° or more (aortic dissection in type-4 Ehlers–Danlos syndrome). (Reprinted with permission from Elsevier. Copyright 1997) (Reference*: Wynne-Davis R. Acetabular dysplasia and familial joint laxity: two etiologic factors in congenital dislocation of the hip. A review of 589 patients and their families. *J Bone Joint Surg* 1970; 52B: 704–716.)

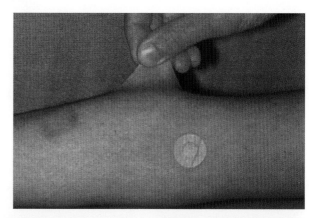

Figure 96 Ehlers–Danlos syndrome: the skin is hyperextensible. The "India rubber man" of circus fame had hyperextensible joints and skin. (Reprinted with permission from Elsevier. Copyright 1997)

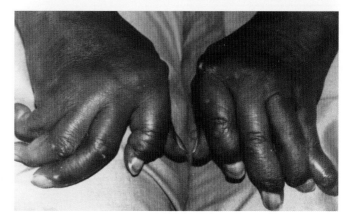

Figure 97 Rheumatoid arthritis of hands: same patient as in Figure 48. The metacarpophalangeal joints are swollen and show marked ulnar deviation (premature CAD). (Reprinted with permission from Humana Press. Copyright 2006)

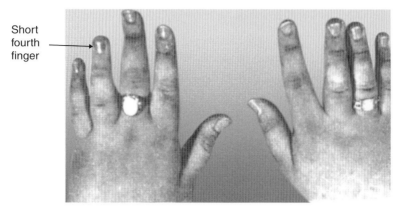

Short
fourth
finger

Figure 98 Short fourth fingers in a patient with Turner syndrome. Same patient as in Figure 11. (Copyright 2003. McGraw Hill. All rights reserved)

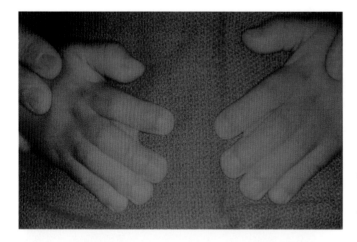

Figure 99 Syndactyly: webbing is clearly seen between index and middle fingers as well as between fingers 3–4 and 4–5 (Prolonged Q-T syndrome). (Reprinted with permission from Elsevier. Copyright 1995)

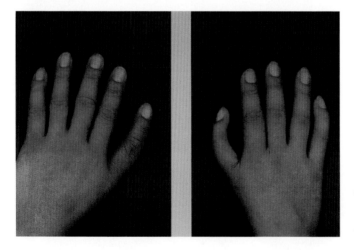

Figure 100 Holt–Oram syndrome: a 29-year-old woman whose left hand shows a thumb with an extra phalanx and resembles a finger. The right hand also shows an extra digit in the right thumb which is curved medially. Secundum atrial septal defect. (Copyright 1998. Lippincott, Williams & Wilkins. All rights reserved)

Extra digit

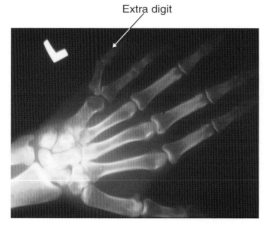

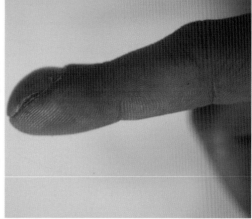

Figure 101 Extra fifth digit is seen on a hand X-ray. A 33-year-old man who had a secundum atrial septal defect.

Figure 104 Clubbing: a profile view of the finger showing an increase in the hyponychial angle and nail-bed angle. The pulp tissue is increased giving the finger a drumstick appearance. Same patient as in Figure 103.

Figure 102 Char syndrome: the fifth middle phalanges are absent, and fifth proximal and distal phalanges are hypoplastic (Persistent ductus arteriosus). (Copyright 1999. Lippincott, Williams & Wilkins. All rights reserved)

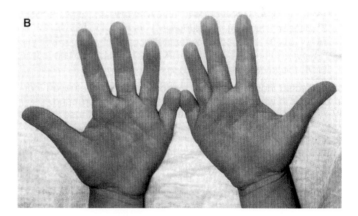

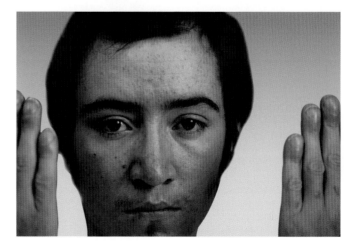

Figure 103 Tetralogy of Fallot: a 22-year-old man with polycythemia, cyanosis, and clubbing.

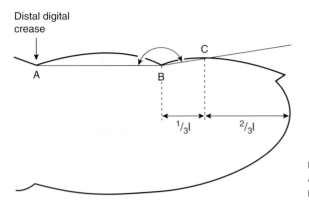

Distal digital crease

Figure 105 The profile nail-bed angle is depicted ABC (normal = 150–170°). (Reprinted with permission from Humana Press. Copyright 2006)

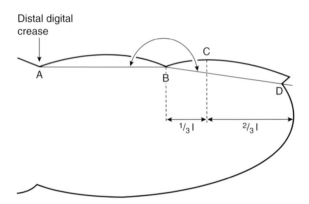

Distal digital crease

Figure 106 The hyponychial nail-bed angle ABD is seen (normal = 178–192°). (Reprinted with permission from Humana Press. Copyright 2006)

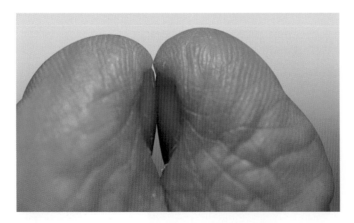

Figure 107 A negative Shamroth sign in a patient without clubbing. There is a narrow slit seen between adjacently placed thumbs.

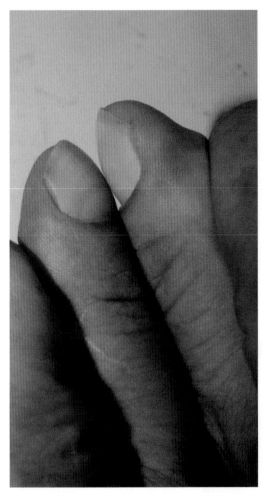

Figure 108 Shamroth sign in a patient with clubbing: there is loss of the normal slit between the two thumbs because of an increase of the hyponychial angle in both the thumbnails.

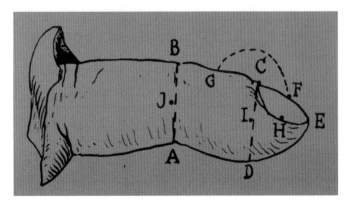

Figure 109 Normal digit in profile showing how to measure the distal phalangeal/interphalangeal depth ratio. AB, distal interphalangeal joint depth; CD, distal phalangeal depth; CD/AB is normally 0.90 with a standard deviation of 0.04.(Copyright 1971. American Thoracic Society. All rights reserved)

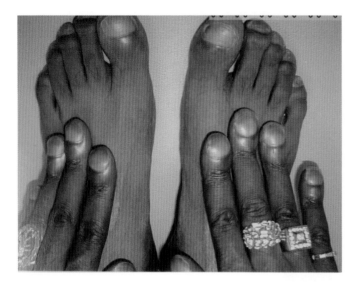

Figure 110 Clubbing of hands and feet in a 25-year-old patient with a right-to-left shunt at the ventricular level. There is subcuticular edema and bulbous appearance of the distal phalanges.

Normal nail bed angle

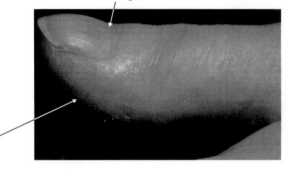

Loss of finger pulp

Figure 111 Nail-bed beaking: this may be mistaken for clubbing, however there is loss of distal tissue pulp and the profile angle is preserved (Copyright 1996. Cliggott Publishing Group. All rights reserved)

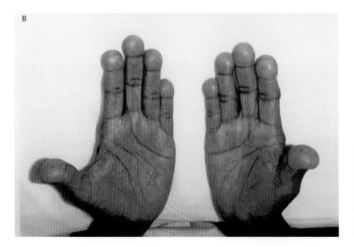

Figure 112 Acro-osteolysis or pseudoclubbing: the distal digits are flattened and bulbous as seen from the palmar side. Nail-bed angle is normal He had secondary hyperparathyroidism. (Copyright 2006. Massachusetts Medical Society. All rights reserved)

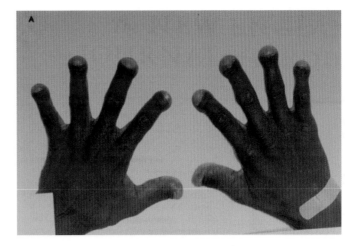

Figure 113 Acro-osteolysis showing the bulbous digits on the dorsal aspect of the hand. The nails are shorter than normal probably due to distal phalangeal subperiosteal resorption. (Copyright 2006. Massachusetts Medical Society. All rights reserved) (Radiographic findings of distal phalangeal resorption are seen in Cheney WD. Acro-osteolysis. *Am J Roentgenol* 1965; 94: 595–607; Figure 1C)

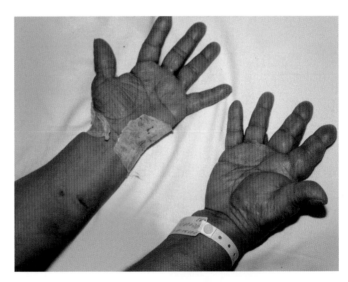

Figure 114 Chronic subclavian vein occlusion: elderly asymptomatic female with mild diabetes. She had painless swelling of the right hand for as long as she can remember.

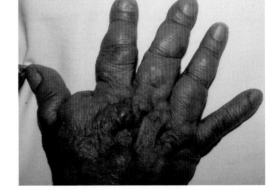

Figure 115 Chronic subclavian vein occlusion. Same patient as in Figure 114. The dorsum of the right hand shows distended veins and cyanotic nail beds. Normal arterial pulses.

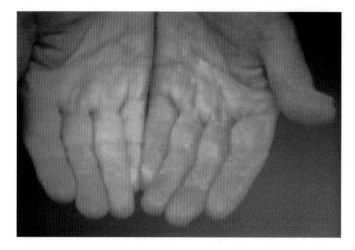

Figure 116 Raynaud's phenomenon: there is pallor of the entire right hand (collagen diseases). Unilateral hand involvement is a rarity. (Source unknown)

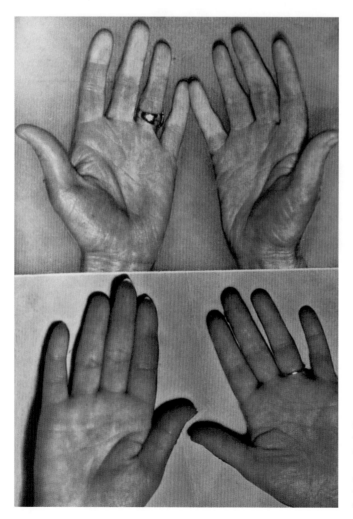

Figure 117 Raynaud's phenomenon. Small areas of pallor are seen in the fingers of both hands when exposed to cold (upper photo). Cyanotic phase at left compared to a normal colored hand on the right (lower photo). (Reprinted with permission from Mayo Clinic. Copyright 1980)

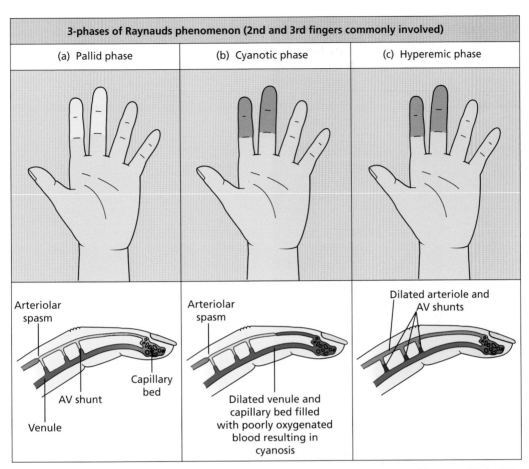

Figure 118 Stages of Raynaud's phenomenon: pallor, then cyanosis, and finally hyperemia. (Based in part on Wigley FM. The differential diagnosis of Raynaud's phenomenon. *Hosp Pract* 1991; 26: 63–70; Figure 2.)

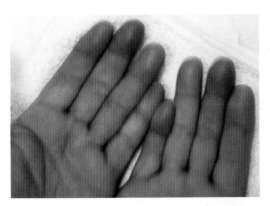

Figure 119 Acrocyanosis: a 35-year-old male with chronic painless cyanosis of several fingertips. Possible collagen vascular disease.

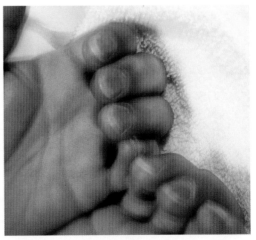

Figure 120 Acrocyanosis: same patient as in Figure 119, showing cyanosis of most of the fingernails.

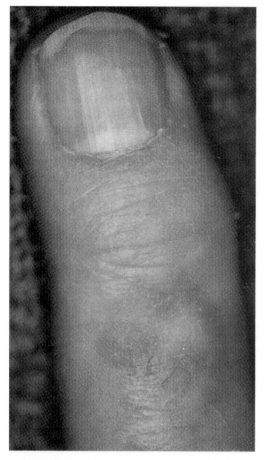

Figure 121 Diagnostician's digit. There is bruising of the middle finger caused by percussion. (Copyright 1997. American Medical Association. All rights reserved)

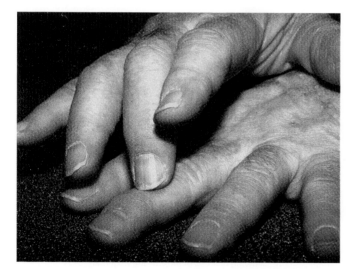

Figure 122 The percussing finger (plexor) has caused bruising of the middle finger (pleximeter) in a physician who has practiced percussion for many years. (Copyright 1997. American Medical Association. All rights reserved)

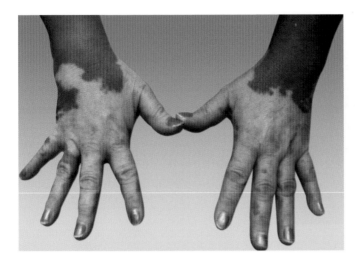

Figure 123 Vitiligo of the forearm and hand. The patient had hyperthyroidism that had been successfully treated 20 years ago.

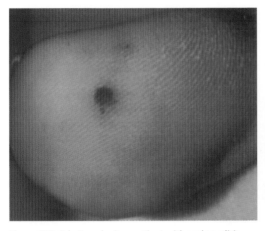

Figure 124 Osler's nodes in a patient with endocarditis: the toe is painful, swollen, and shows a 2-mm-red nodule of the pulp tissue. (Copyright 1982. Mayo Clinic. All rights reserved)

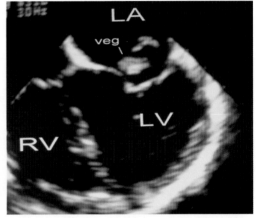

Figure 125 Endocarditis. Transesophageal echocardiogram showing a vegetation on the mitral valve. LA, left atrium; LV, left ventricle; RV, right ventricle; Veg, vegetation.

Figure 126 Endocarditis. Same patient as in Figure 125. On the left, color Doppler study in four-chamber view showing a turbulent systolic jet of mitral regurgitation directed toward the lateral wall of the left atrium. LA, left atrium; LV, left ventricle; *, level of mitral valve; RV, right ventricle. On the right, pulsed Doppler study shows mitral regurgitation jet (MR). E = E point on mitral valve.

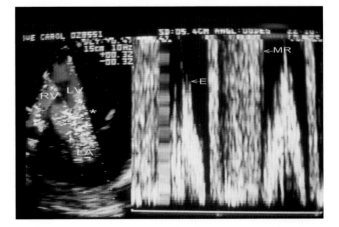

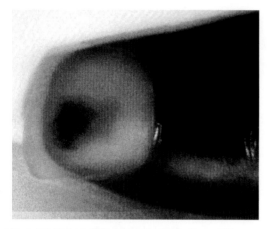

Figure 127 Endocarditis: same patient as in Figure 125. There is a large subungal hemorrhage.

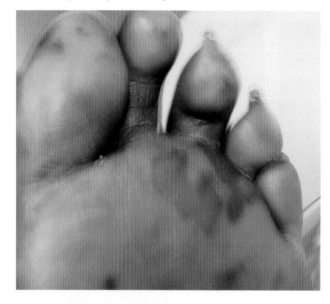

Figure 128 Endocarditis: same patient as in Figure 125. There are dark blue and red patchy areas on the toes and soles of the feet, which are painless. These areas are Janeway lesions. Good peripheral pulses.

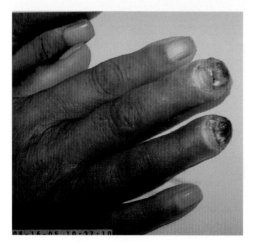

Figure 129 Frostbite and atherosclerotic disease of the hand: a 62-year-old man with three-vessel coronary artery disease, hypertension, and a history of frostbite. His middle and ring fingertips were painful and showed areas of necrosis. Doppler pressure measurements showed a hand/brachial ratio of only 0.6. Six months later his hands were completely healed.

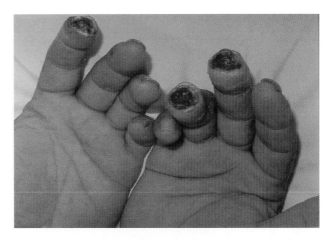

Figure 130 Frostbite of hands from palmar side. Same patient as in Figure 129.

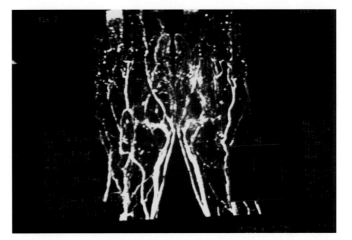

Figure 131 MRA of hand of patient (Figure 130) showing extensive collateral circulation and occlusive arterial disease of the hand. The palmar arches (deep and superficial) are not seen.

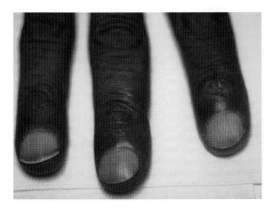

Figure 132 White nails in a patient with chronic hepatic congestion secondary to heart failure.

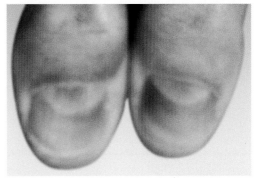

Figure 133 Red lunulae in a patient with heart failure.

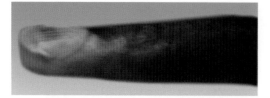

Figure 134 Plummer's nails in a patient with hyperthyroidism (same patient as in Figure 35). The brown discoloration is dirt that has penetrated half way under the nail bed because of onycholysis.

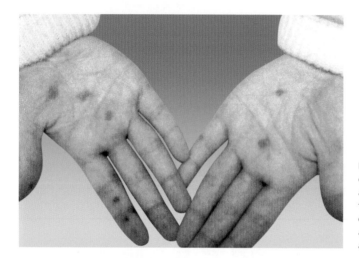

Figure 135 Palmar lesions simulating endocarditis with peripheral emboli or a vasculitis in a 34-year-old Korean female with peripartum cardiomyopathy who was on Coumadin and had acupuncture of the hands in an attempt to alleviate her dyspnea.

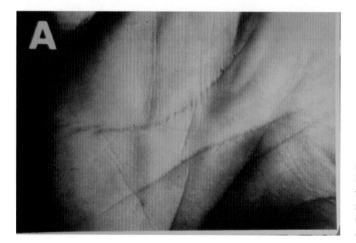

Figure 136 Type-3 broad beta hyperlipidemia. There is yellowing of the palmar creases also referred to as xanthochromia striatum palmaris. (Copyright 1983. *Annals of Internal Medicine*. All rights reserved)

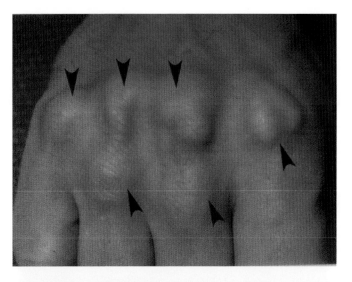

Figure 137 Tendon xanthoma of knuckles. Serum cholesterol 460 mg/dL.

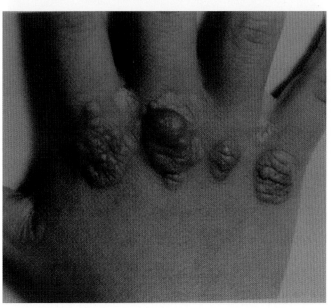

Figure 138 Tuberous xanthoma of interdigital area. Serum cholesterol 1120 mg/dL.

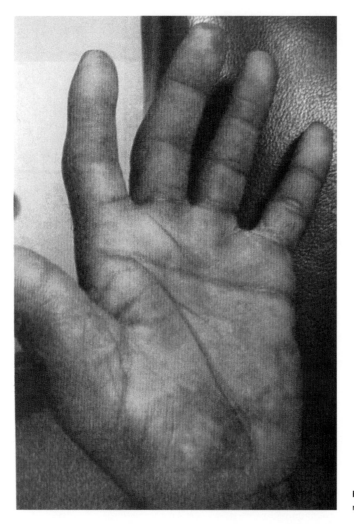

Figure 139 Simian crease seen in a normal subject.

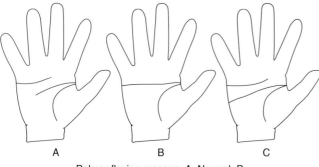

Palmar flexion creases. A. Normal. B. Simian crease. C. sydney line.

Figure 140 Palmar creases in normals and Down syndrome: (a) normal; (b) Simian crease; (c) Sydney line. In (b), the proximal transverse crease is long and extends to the ulnar side of the palm; and the distal transverse crease is absent. In (c), the distal palmar crease is present and the proximal transverse crease extends to the ulnar side of the palm. (b) and (c) may occur in Down syndrome.

CHAPTER 7

Upper extremity

Stretch marks over the shoulders and upper chest may suggest rapid weight change, but can also be seen in weight lifters. Venous tracks due to IV drug abuse are usually seen on the forearms (Figure 141—same patient as seen in Figure 17). There may be a surgical scar in the antecubital fossa from a previous cardiac catheterization or one along the radial artery (Figure 142) if it was required for aortocoronary artery bypass grafting.

An AV fistula may be seen in the arm in patients requiring chronic hemodialysis (Figure 143 and 144).

In disseminated lupus erythematosus there may be red discrete papular or urticarial lesions on the arms (Figure 145). The patient depicted in Figure 145 had also a malar butterfly skin eruption. Derma-tomyositis may show violaceous, discrete scaly papular eruptions usually on the arms. A proximal myopathy is often seen in dermatomyositis [42]. Tuberous xanthomas occur on the elbow and reflect an elevated cholesterol level (Figure 146) [187]. Eruptive xanthomas occur in crops on the arms, back, and buttocks and indicate an elevated triglyceride level (Figure 166). Hypertriglyceridemia is a coronary artery risk factor [188].

Coumadin-induced skin necrosis can occur in the arms (Figure 147) [189] but usually occurs in the legs or thighs (Figure 148). Protein C levels are reduced.

Heparin-induced skin necrosis may be seen in the arms and is attributed to a hypersensitivity angiitis (Figure 149) [190].

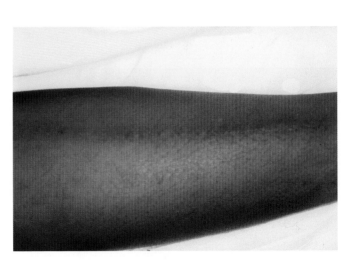

Figure 141 Venous track in a heroin addict (same patient as in Figure 17).

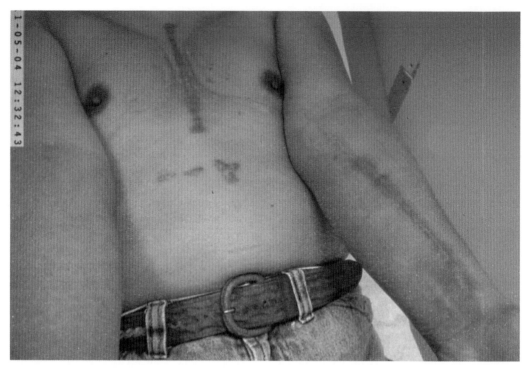

Figure 142 Radial artery scar. The patient had undergone coronary artery bypass surgery in which the left radial artery was harvested. He also had a median sternotomy scar.

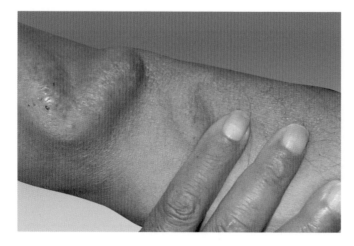

Figure 143 Arteriovenous fistula in a patient undergoing chronic renal dialysis. He has white nails probably due to a low serum albumin.

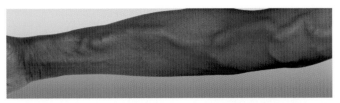

Figure 144 An extensive arteriovenous fistula in another renal dialysis patient involving forearm and arm. Continuous bruit was best heard over the forearm.

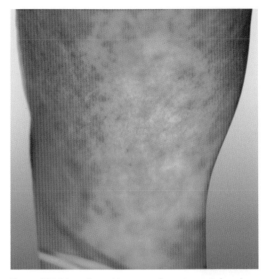

Figure 145 Disseminated lupus erythematosus. A female with discrete papular lesions over the forearm. She also had a butterfly malar eruption.

Figure 146 Tuberous xanthoma: yellow nodules are noted over the elbow. (Copyright 1994. American Medical Association. All rights reserved)

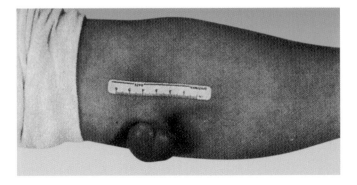

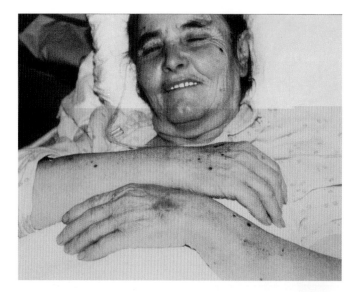

Figure 147 Coumadin-induced skin necrosis of hands. The patient shows patchy areas of red mottling (hemorrhage under the skin) and dark red macules representing areas of possible necrosis. (Copyright 1998. Cliggott Publishing Group. All rights reserved)

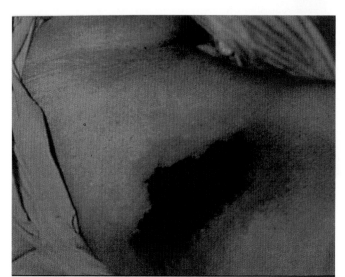

Figure 148 More extensive area of Coumadin skin necrosis of thigh. (Reprinted with permission from Elsevier. Copyright 1997)

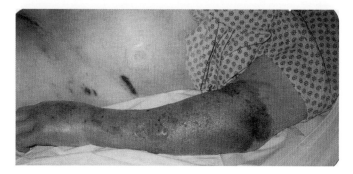

Figure 149 Heparin-induced skin necrosis of forearm and thorax. The arm is diffusely red and swollen. In addition, there are areas of ecchymosis and bullae. (Copyright 1998. Resident and Staff Physician. All rights reserved)

CHAPTER 8

Thorax and back

The thorax and back should be examined for visible pulsations, presence or absence of a sternal hump, prominent vessels on the chest wall, surgical incisions, chest wall deformities, and skin lesions [heparin-induced thrombocytopenic purpura (HIT), lentigines, gynecomastia, neurofibroma, eruptive xanthoma, and radiation effects].

The proper evaluation of precordial pulsations requires the combined use of inspection, palpation, and/or auscultation [191]. Only a summary of the diagnostic value of those readily visible precordial pulsations, listed by location is given here:

- *Sternoclavicular joints*: Aortic regurgitation, aortic aneurysm, dissecting aneurysm.
- *Right second interspace parasternally*: Dilated ascending aorta due to either aortic regurgitation or aortic aneurysm.
- *Second or third left interspace parasternally*: Pulmonary hypertension or an increase in pulmonary blood flow.
- *Left lower sternal border*: Right ventricular enlargement or hypertrophy of any cause.

Moderate to severe mitral regurgitation may produce a late systolic lift.

- *Between left lower sternal border and apex*: Aneurysm of the anterior wall of the left ventricle.
- *Apical area*: Normally the apex beat is in fifth interspace, no more than 10 cm from the mid sternal line in an adult without any chest wall deformity [191]. Cardiomegaly may be detected if the apex beat is greater than 10 cm from the mid sternal line in the fifth (or lower) interspace. Detection of the size and character of the apex beat is also important. This requires a combination of palpation and/or auscultation and has been discussed elsewhere [191]. Inspection of the back may reveal intercostal pulsations due to collateral arteries, which are often seen in coarctation of the aorta.

A sternal hump or mass is usually of inflammatory or neoplastic origin [192]. It is very rarely due to an ascending aortic aneurysm eroding the sternum. It was not uncommon in the past to see a pulsatile sternal mass due to a syphilitic aortic aneurysm eroding the chest wall (Figure 150).

The presence of venous stars [193] on the anterior chest wall is a feature of the superior vena cava syndrome. Other features (Figures 151–156) of the superior vena cava syndrome include unilateral neck vein distention, prominent venous collaterals over the chest wall, suffusion of face, and retinal vein engorgement [83].[5] Scars of various surgical procedures should also be noted, e.g., median sternotomy, lateral thoracotomy, tracheostomy, mediastinoscopy, pacemaker or implantable defibrillator insertion sites, and port-a-cath placement (Figure 157).

The normal transverse diameter/(anterior–posterior diameter) ratio of the chest is 1.4:1 in youth [194] and 1.0 in old age.

Deformities of the spine or rib cage [195, 196] may also provide a clue to the presence of cardiovascular disease (Figures 158 and 159).

1 A patient is defined as having a straight back syndrome when the transverse diameter/anteroposterior diameter is over 3 and there is loss of the normal dorsal kyphosis [197]. Such patients may have a pulmonary flow murmur without pulmonic stenosis or an ASD [196, 197] (Figure 159).
2 A shield chest is a broad chest with widely spaced nipples and an increased angle between manubrium

---

[5] An ancient Greek statue "the old fisherman" depicts an example of advanced superior vena cava syndrome with prominent venous collaterals on the chest wall (The Louvre Museum, Paris) (Figure 151).

and the body of the sternum. It is seen in Turner syndrome (Figure 11) and LEOPARD syndrome (Figure 20).

3 Pectus carinatum (pigeon chest) is associated with Marfan syndrome (Figure 158).

4 Pectus excavatum is seen in Marfan syndrome, Noonan's syndrome, homocystinuria, Ehlers–Danlos syndrome, and gargoylism.

5 A bamboo spine (Figures 160 and 161) is seen in ankylosing spondylitis (aortic regurgitation, mitral regurgitation, cardiomyopathy) [198]. In milder cases, there is limited separation of the spinous processes on bending down (Schober test).

6 Kyphoscoliosis may give rise to cor pulmonale. Kyphoscoliosis occurs in Friedriech's ataxia, Hurler's syndrome, Marfan syndrome (Figure 158) neurofibromatosis, and adults with William's syndrome [199].

7 Deep sternal wound infections (0.47% seen in patients who underwent open heart surgery) [200] may occasionally require a sternectomy. The heart then bulges out of the chest cavity, covered only by a thin layer of grafted skin (Figure 162).

Note: A barrel-shaped chest (defined as a transverse/AP diameter of 1.0) (Figure 163) is an unreliable sign of chronic obstructive lung disease as it has also been found in the elderly patient without chronic obstructive lung disease [194].

HIT may be seen on the chest wall (Figure 164), but may involve in any part of the body.

Lentigines are seen in the LEOPARD syndrome (Figure 52) [60]. Gynecomastia is seen in hyperestrogenism and patients on digitalis or aldosterone [201].

Neurofibromatosis (von Reckinghausen's disease) occurs in 1:3000 of the population and may be associated with hypertension due to the coexistent pheochromocytoma or renal artery disease [202]. Cardiac neurofibromas may produce outflow tract obstruction [203].

The skin lesions of neurofibromatosis (café au lait macules over 1.5 cm in diameter, neurofibromas, axillary, or inguinal freckling) are randomly distributed, but occur often on the chest or back (Figure 165).

Eruptive xanthomas may also occur on the back or the gluteal area. They are seen in patients with hypertriglyceridemia (Figure 166).

Patient receiving extensive radiation therapy to the mediastinum or abdomen some years previously may show atrophy of the paravertebral muscles (Figure 167) [204, 205] and chronic radiation dermatitis (skin atrophy, pigmentary changes, and telangiectasia). Radiotherapy of the mediastinum may give rise to coronary artery stenosis, pericarditis, myocarditis [206, 207], or aortic regurgitation [208].

Excessive radiation from repeated coronary angioplasties or a prolonged electrophysiologic study may produce chronic nonhealing ulcers of the back (Figure 168) [209].

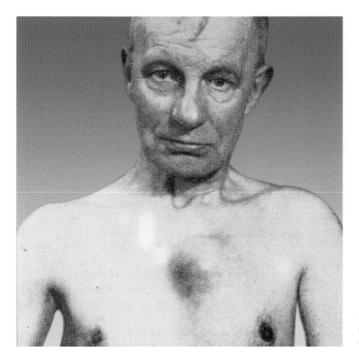

Figure 150 Luetic aortitis: an ascending aortic aneurysm is eroding the anterior chest wall. (Reprinted with permission from Hodder. Copyright 1960)

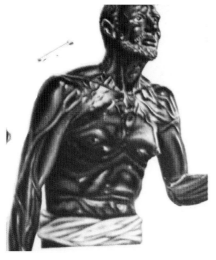

Figure 151 Superior vena cava syndrome. This Roman sculpture entitled The Old Fisherman shows extensive venous collateral circulation over the chest wall as well as distended arm veins.

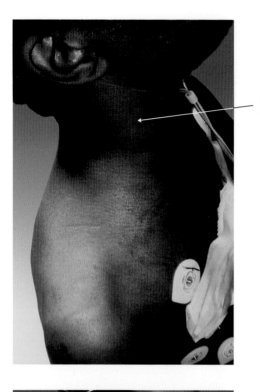

Distended
neck vein

Figure 152 Superior vena cava syndrome: the
right jugular vein is distended and less
flagrant venous collaterals are see over the
right upper chest as compared to Figure 151.

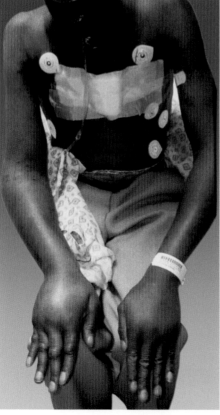

Figure 153 Superior vena cava syndrome: there is asymmetric
swelling of the hands. Same patient as in Figure 152. He had
lung cancer obstructing the superior vena cava.

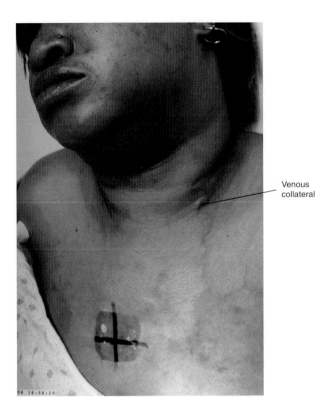

Venous
collateral

Figure 154 Superior vena cava syndrome: a 48-year-old female showing some left neck vein distention and prominent venous collateral circulation over the left upper chest. She is receiving radiation therapy at point X for small cell carcinoma of lung. She had some facial swelling.

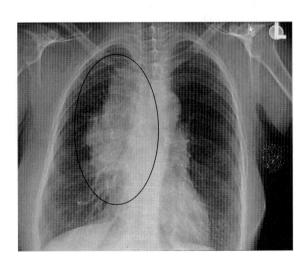

Figure 155 Superior vena cava syndrome: Same patient as in Figure 154, showing an extensive right hilar and paratracheal mass on chest X-ray.

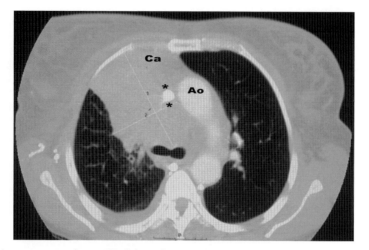

Figure 156 Superior vena cava syndrome: C/T of chest of same patient as in Figure 154, showing compression of superior vena cava (between * *) by a mass as well as subcutaneous edema. Ao, aorta; Ca, lung cancer.

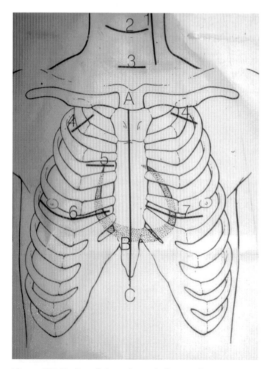

Figure 157 Neck and thoracic surgical scars of cardiovascular importance 1, carotid endarterectomy; 2, thyroid surgery; 3, tracheostomy or mediastinoscopy; 4, pacemaker, implantable defibrillator; 5, port-a-cath site; 6, right-sided thoracotomy; 7, minimally invasive coronary artery bypass surgery. ABC, median sternotomy; BC, pericardial window.

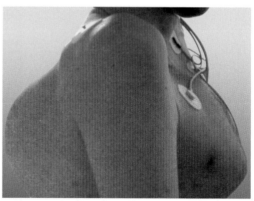

Figure 158 Kyphoscoliosis and pectus carinatum: a 44-year-old man with Marfan syndrome. He had been operated upon at age 38 for dissecting aneurysm of the aorta.

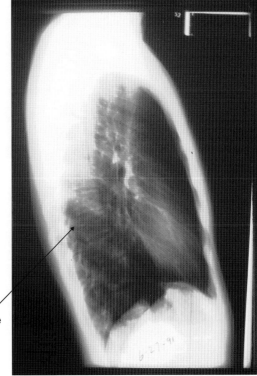

Loss of
normal
thoracic
curvature

Figure 159 Chest Roentgenogram—lateral view—a 30-year-old male showing straight back syndrome. He had loss of normal dorsal kyphosis.

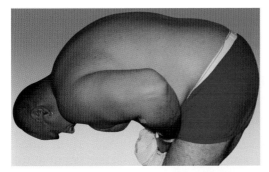

Figure 160 Ankylosing spondylitis: a 40-year-old man admitted with heart failure (left ventricular ejection fraction 26%). No history of alcoholism or smoking. Chest expansion was only 2 cm. Schober test showed only 0.5 cm increase in L1–L5 distance on bending down.

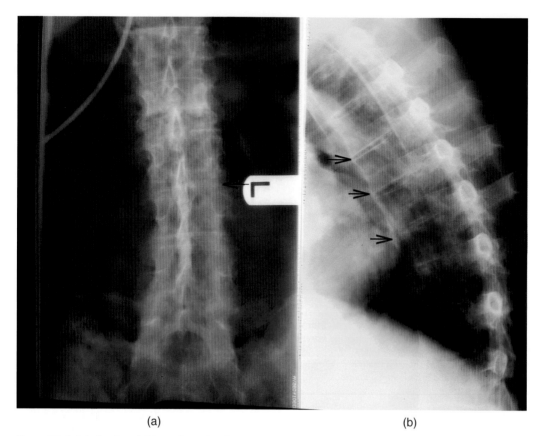

(a)   (b)

Figure 161 Ankylosing Spondylitis. Radiographs of patient in Figure 160. a) Lumbosacral spine showing ossification of the spinal ligaments and narrowing of the intervertebral spaces to create a bamboo spine appearance. The sacro-iliac joint is sclerosed and b) Oblique view of Thoracic spine showing bony bridging between the thoracic vertebrae (arrows)

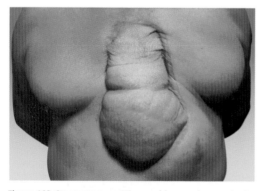

Figure 162 Sternectomy: a 60-year-old man who required a sternectomy after a sternal wound infection following cardiac transplantation 11 years ago. The heart is bulging out of the thoracic cage covered by a thin layer of skin. The patient is obliged to wear a chest shield when he drives.

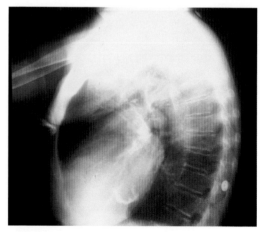

Figure 163 Chest roentgenogram—lateral view—a 90-year-old man with marked kyphosis, appearing as a barrel shaped chest. Mitral annular calcification is also seen.

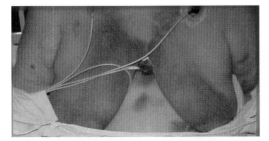

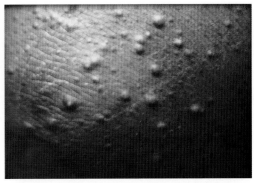

Figure 164 Heparin induced thrombocytopenia: an 80-year-old female developed an extensive area of ecchymosis over the anterior chest wall and severe thrombocytopenia. Four days previously, she had sustained an acute myocardial infarction, receiving heparin and requiring DC shock to the chest wall for ventricular tachycardia. She had received heparin in the past for a deep vein thrombosis without any ill effects. Heparin was stopped and the ecchymosis on the chest wall cleared up within 4 weeks. (Reprinted with permission from Human Press. Copyright 2006)

Figure 166 Eruptive xanthoma of back: this patient had discrete papules with a yellow center resembling acne vulgaris. Triglyceride level >2000 mg/dL. (Reprinted with permission from Human Press. Copyright 2006)

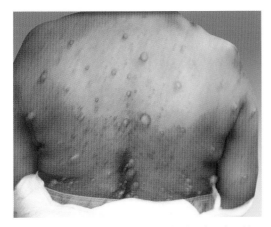

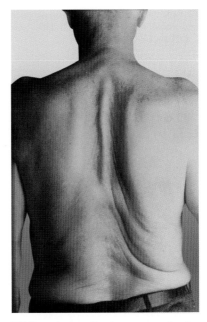

Figure 165 Neurofibromatosis of the back: a female with brown papules and brown soft pedunculated nodules are seen over the back and arms. She also had several café au lait macules on the arms (not shown) (hypertension, cardiac tumors).

Figure 167 Paraspinal wasting is seen, secondary to radiation of the mediastinum (coronary artery disease). (Copyright 2000. Cliggott Publishing Group. All rights reserved)

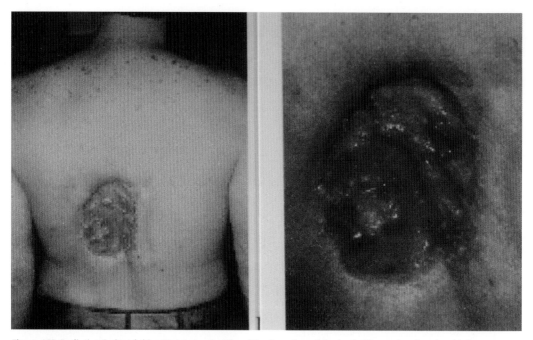

Figure 168 Radiation-induced skin necrosis: nonhealing skin ulceration of the back, 22 months after the third coronary angioplasty procedure. Closeup view on right showing tissue necrosis. (Copyright 1996. Radiological Society of North America. All rights reserved)

9

CHAPTER 9

Abdomen

While Cullen's sign and Gray–Turner's sign are typically seen in hemorrhagic pancreatitis [210], these signs are also seen in retroperitoneal bleeding caused by anticoagulants (Figures 169 and 170), post-lithotripsy (Figures 171–173), or a leaking abdominal aortic stent.

A rectus sheath hematoma may occur as a result of injury to the epigastric artery following a bout of severe coughing. Cherry and Mueller [211] noted that such patients are usually over 68 years old and are on anticoagulants. These patients develop severe diffuse abdominal pain, an abdominal mass, and extensive abdominal wall ecchymoses (Figures 174 and 175).

Reddish striae may occur on the lateral wall of the abdomen in Cushing's syndrome (hypertension) (Figure 176).

Angiokeratomas (punctuate dark blue or red or black nonblanching macules) may be seen between the umbilicus and the thighs ("swimming trunk area") in Fabry's disease (Figures 177 and 178).

Fabry's disease is a rare X-linked recessive lysosomal storage disorder in which there is a deficiency of alpha-galactosidase A, resulting in the deposition of glycosphingolipids in the vascular endothelium. Widespread vascular occlusive disease then occurs which results in CAD, cerebral arterial thrombosis, and renal failure [212].

Distended superficial anterolateral abdominal veins are seen in inferior vena cava obstruction (Figure 179) [213]. These veins when emptied by applying the two index fingers 3–5 cm apart, fill from below when the pressure is released by the inferiorly placed finger.

Hepatomegaly is seen in heart failure, Wilson's disease, hemochromatosis, or chronic alcoholism. Ascites is seen in right heart failure, tricuspid valve disease, and constrictive pericarditis [214]. Cardiac ascites accounts for only 5% of all causes of ascites [214].

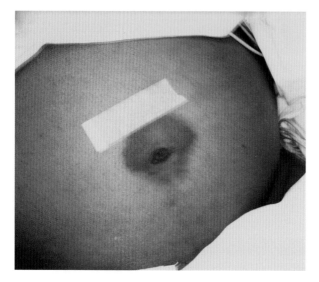

Figure 169 Cullen's sign: this patient developed a periumbilical ecchymosis associated with Coumadin overdose. Prothrombin time was 110 seconds. (Reprinted with permission from Human Press. Copyright 2006)

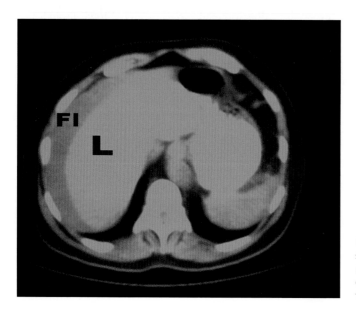

Figure 170 CAT scan of the abdomen showed fluid around the liver (same patient as in Figure 169) presumably due to retroperitoneal bleeding. L, liver; fl, fluid.

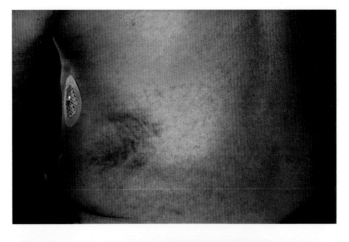

Figure 171 Gray–Turner's sign: a 70-year-old man who developed an area of ecchymosis of the left flank following a left renal lithotripsy.

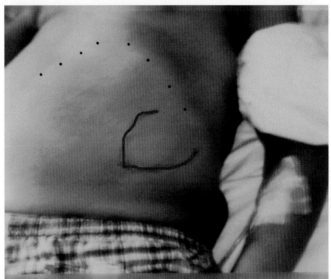

Figure 172 The left kidney is enlarged and palpable as marked on abdomen. Same patient as in Figure 171.

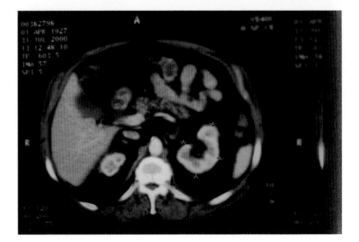

Figure 173 CAT scan of abdomen of same patient (Figure 171) showing a large perinephric hematoma involving the left kidney (surrounded by ***).

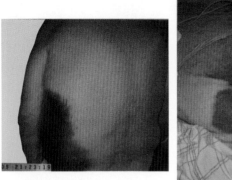

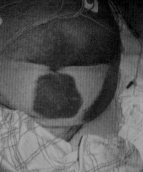

Figure 174 Rectus sheath hematoma: a 75-year-old man admitted with severe abdominal pain following a coughing spell. He had an extensive hematoma over the abdomen. He was on Coumadin for atrial fibrillation. PT/INR was 3. Hemoglobin fell to 8 g%. After treating the patient with blood transfusion, analgesics, and stopping Coumadin the abdominal hematoma gradually faded over the next 2 weeks.

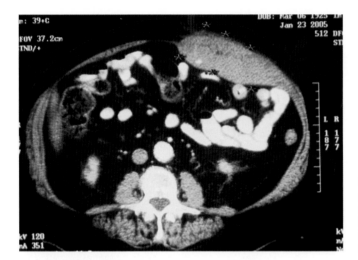

Figure 175 CAT scan of abdomen of patient above showed a right-sided rectus sheath hematoma (encompassed by ***) resembling a snake's head and body. The left rectus muscle is uniformly thin.

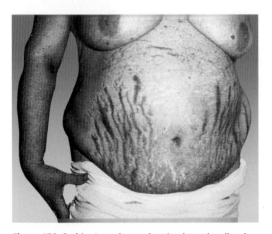

Figure 176 Cushing's syndrome showing lateral wall red striae (hypertension). (Reprinted with permission from Elsevier. Copyright 1998)

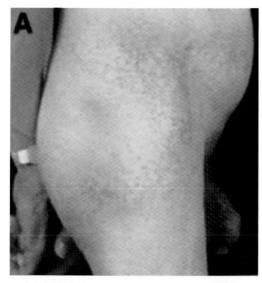

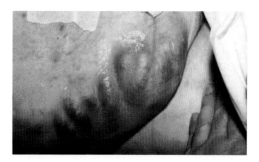

Figure 179 Inferior vena cava obstruction: there are prominent collateral veins coursing over the anterior and lateral abdominal wall. The abdominal wall is edematous. (Copyright 1991. Cliggott Publishing Group. All rights reserved)

Figure 177 Fabry's disease: Angiokeratoma are seen, distributed between the umbilicus and the upper thigh, consisting of numerous dark red lesions ranging in size from pinhead to several millimeters in diameter. These lesions are nonblanching and become larger and more numerous with age. (Copyright 2003. Annals of Internal Medicine. All rights reserved)

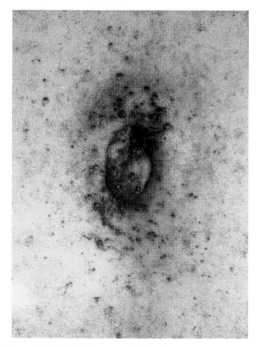

Figure 178 Fabry's disease: angiokeratomas are seen around the umbilicus. (Copyright 2003. Annals of Internal Medicine. All rights reserved)

CHAPTER 10

Lower extremity

The lower extremity should be examined for edema. Bilateral leg edema is seen in heart failure, severe tricuspid regurgitation, chronic constrictive pericarditis, venous insufficiency, venous thrombosis, hypoalbuminemia, or severe anemia. Of the causes of bilateral leg edema, only heart failure is associated with an elevated jugular venous pressure.

Unilateral leg edema is suggestive of local venous obstruction (Figure 180).

Lymphedema, phlebitis (Figure 181), and arterial occlusive disease (Figures 182–184) are well described elsewhere [215, 216].

Erythema nodosum consists of red tender subcutaneous nodular eruptions, 1–5 mm in diameter, that are usually found over the extensor surfaces of the legs [217] (Figure 185). Sarcoidosis is one of the commoner causes of erythema nodosum [217], which in turn is associated with ventricular arrhythmias, complete heart block, and cor pulmonale.

Erythema marginatum is a pink circular eruption with a pale center and raised margins that is usually seen on the trunk, limbs, or axillae. It is most commonly due to rheumatic fever and occurs in 25% of cases [218]. It usually precedes joint involvement and the appearance of carditis and is a major criterion for rheumatic fever. While rare in the West (5:100,000), it is more common in the developing countries (100–1000:100,000) [218] (Figure 186).

Skin popping sites are rounded scars, 1–3 cm in diameter, seen on the legs and arms of drug abusers who inject heroin subcutaneously (Figures 187 and 188). Extensive cellulitis and scarring of the thighs occur with repeated subcutaneous injections of heroin/cocaine (Figure 189). Janeway lesions are usually seen on the soles of the feet (Figure 190) and are a feature of endocarditis [175].

Subungal fibromas may be seen in the feet and are suggestive of tuberous sclerosis (Figure 62 and 63) [67, 69]. Buerger's disease (Figures 191 and 192) is a nonatherosclerotic inflammatory obliterative disease characterized by thrombotic occlusion of the small- and median-sized vessels of the lower extremities, and less commonly the upper extremities. Gangrene of one or more digits may occur. Buerger's disease has usually been regarded as occurring mostly in males <40 years of age who are heavy smokers. Recent studies [176] show that Buerger's disease is now more common in the 40–60 age groups and that the male/female ratio has dropped from 9/1 to 3/1. Thirty percent of patients have an associated superficial thrombophlebitis [176].

In diabetic vasculopathy, there is initially an impalpable foot pulse and then a single blue toe, which becomes gangrenous. Purple toe syndrome, however, is characterized by multiple bluish red toes and palpable arterial pulses (Figure 193). It is caused by atheromatous emboli (which also contains cholesterol) originating from the abdominal aorta [219–221]. Patients with frostbite may have several gangrenous toes and impalpable pulses (Figure 194).

Livedo reticularis is an erythematous pruritic macular eruption resembling the imprint of fine mesh wiring on the skin. It typically occurs on the feet and is due to atheromatous emboli following surgical manipulation of the aorta [222]. The foot pulses are preserved.

Xanthomas are infiltrates containing lipid-filled histiocytes deposited in either the dermis or tendons. They are yellow because of their carotene content. Xanthomas are seen in hyperlipidemias as follows:

(a) *Hypercholesterolemia*: Tuberous xanthomas are flat or elevated yellow nodules seen mainly on the knees (Figure 195) or elbows (Figure 146). Tendon xanthomas are yellow papules or nodules found on the patella tendon (Figure 196) dorsum of the feet or tendo Achilles. They may also occur on the dorsum of the hand [223] (Figure 137).

(b) *Hypertriglyceridemia*: Eruptive xanthomas usually occur when the plasma triglyceride is 1000–2000 mg% [224]. They are discrete yellow papular lesions surrounded by an erythematous base and most commonly found on the buttock, back, elbows, and knees. At this stage these lesions may be mistaken for acne. They appear suddenly in crops and may coalesce to form plaques (tuberous xanthoma). In the example (Figure 197), the patient had a triglyceride level of 3000 mg% and milky white serum (Figure 198). The serum is milky white when the triglycerides are over 600 mg% [225]. Lipemia retinalis may be detected if the plasma triglyceride is over 3000 mg% [226] (Figure 31).

Clubbing of the feet may be seen in cyanotic heart disease. It may be more obvious in the feet than in the hands in the Eisenmenger syndrome (differential clubbing). Pes cavus[6] is a feature of Friedriech's ataxia (Figure 199) (cardiomyopathy) [14].

Pseudohypertrophy of the calf muscles is seen in Duchenne dystrophy which is associated with atrial arrhythmias and regional left ventricular dysfunction [62] (Figure 200). Acute gouty arthritis of the great toe may be seen in patients on thiazide diuretics (Figure 201). Pretibial myxedema occurs in 5% of cases of hyperthyroidism. The skin lesions occur on the legs and dorsa of the feet. These lesions consist of bilateral asymmetric nodules or plaques that give a peau d'orange appearance. When these nodules coalesce, the skin is no longer smooth but takes on a craggy appearance [227].

Saber shins, complaints of increasing hat size, and kyphosis are features of Paget's disease of the bone (high output failure) (Figure 12) [10].

Keratoderma blennorrhagica (Figure 202) is a feature of Reiter's syndrome (conjunctivitis, arthritis, urethritis) occurring in 60% of cases [188]. Keratoderma blennorrhagica occur usually on the soles of the feet or the palms of the hand in white males. They appear as red macules that become hyperkeratotic waxy papules with a central zone of yellow surrounded by a red halo. The papules coalesce to form plaques with subsequent crusting. Aortic regurgitation may occur in 60% of cases of Reiter's syndrome [228].

---

[6]An acquired form of pes cavus was seen in the past from childhood foot binding. It was prevalent in China (T'ang Dynasty until 1911) and in Kutchin Indians from Alaska (Encyclopedia Britannica).

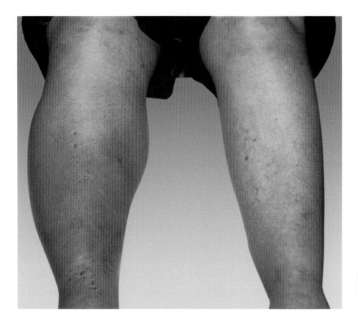

Figure 180 Unilateral swelling of right leg due to venous insufficiency and local cellulitis.

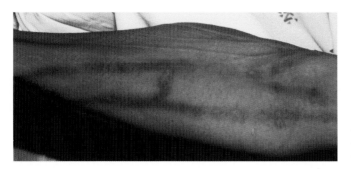

Figure 181 Chemical phlebitis: this patient had received 5-fluorouracil into the arm veins and developed sclerosis of the veins that could be mistaken for the venous tracks of an IV drug addict.

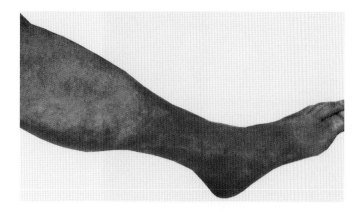

Figure 182 Arterial occlusive disease: a 70-year-old man with new onset of painful bluish mottling of the left leg.

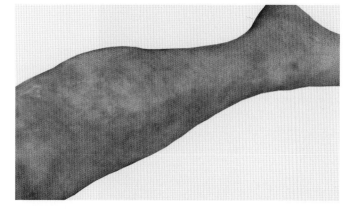

Figure 183 Same patient as in Figure 182, showing painful bluish mottling of right leg.

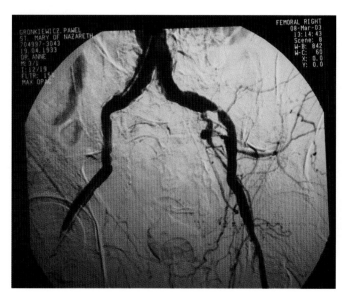

Figure 184 Arteriogram of patient in Figure 182: there is occlusion of the right femoral artery and high-grade stenoses of the left ileofemoral system.

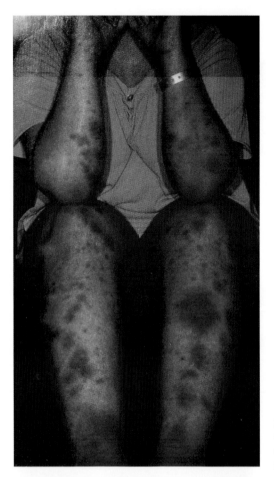

Figure 185 Erythema nodosum: the extensor surface of the legs shows several discrete subcutaneous nodules that are red and painful (Sarcoidosis). (Reprinted with permission from Elsevier. Copyright 1997)

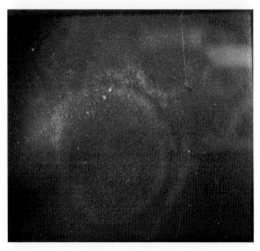

Figure 186 Erythema marginatum: a pink area surrounded by a raised margin seen on the buttocks or thighs (Rheumatic fever). (Copyright 1992. American Medical Association. All rights reserved)

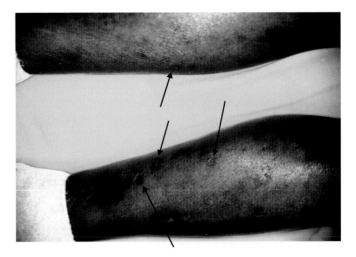

Figure 187 Skin popping sites arrows in the leg where a heroin/cocaine addict would inject the drug under the skin (African American female).

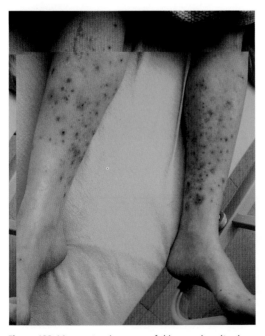

Figure 188 More extensive areas of skin popping sites in a Caucasian drug addict.

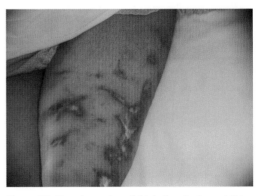

Figure 189 Chronic scarring of thigh: female drug addict who injected heroin subcutaneously into the thigh.

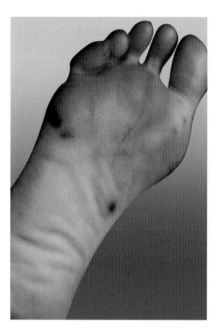

Figure 190 Janeway lesion of the foot: a 40-year-old heroin addict with endocarditis of her mitral and aortic valves. There are painless small red papules on the soles of the feet. (Reprinted with permission from Human Press. Copyright 2006)

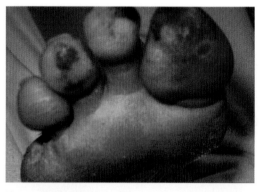

Figure 192 Closeup view of the same patient as in Figure 191, showing necrosis of the toes and cyanosis of right foot.

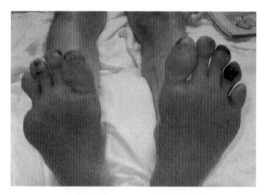

Figure 191 Buerger's disease of the lower extremity. There are asymmetric cyanotic and necrotic changes of the toes. The fifth toe on the right has been amputated for gangrene. This 60-year-old man was a heavy smoker.

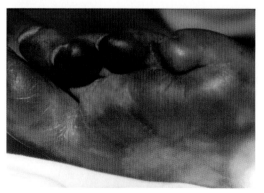

Figure 193 Purple toe syndrome: there is symmetrical purpuric areas involving the toes. The patient had cholesterol emboli. The arterial pulses were palpable.

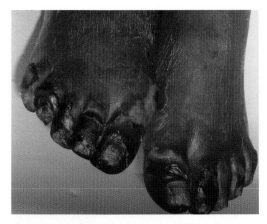

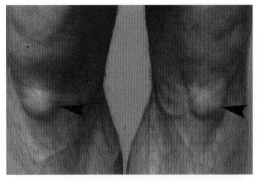

Figure 196 Tendon xanthomas: there are yellow nodules on the patella tendon. Serum cholesterol 460 mg/dL. (Copyright 2002. Annals of Internal Medicine. All rights reserved)

Figure 194 Frostbite of feet: a 50-year-old homeless female who has extensive gangrene of feet. Pulseless and painless feet.

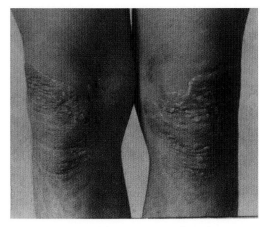

Figure 195 Planar xanthomas: there are flat yellow plaques on the knees (hypercholesterolemia). (Copyright 1994. American Medical Association. All rights reserved)

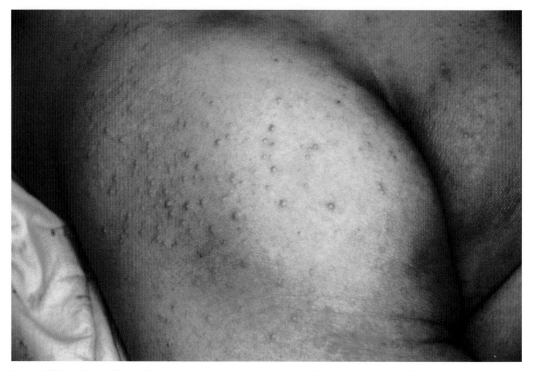

Figure 197 Eruptive xanthoma: there are discrete pink papules with a yellow center and a red rim on the buttocks. Serum triglycerides 3000 mg/dL.

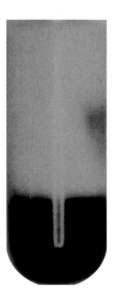

Figure 198 Same patient as in Figure 197. The serum is milky white.

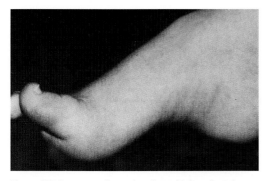

Figure 199 Pes cavus: the patient has a high arch and a hammer great toe (Friedriech's ataxia-cardiomyopathy). (Reprinted with permission from Elsevier. Copyright 1986)

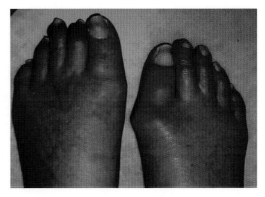

Figure 201 Gout: there is redness, swelling, and pain in the right great toe due to hydrochlorothiazide.

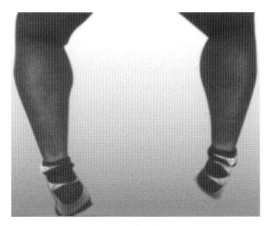

Figure 200 Duchenne dystrophy: there is pseudohypertrophy of the calf muscles. There is an associated waddling gait (LV dysfunction). (Reprinted with permission from Elsevier. Copyright 1986)

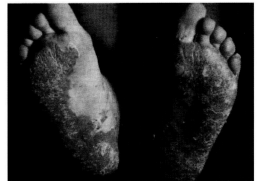

Figure 202 Keratoderma blennorrhagicum: the soles of the feet show hyperkeratotic waxy papules and crusting (aortic regurgitation). (Copyright 1992. Mayo Clinic. All rights reserved)

Appendix: Rarer syndromes associated with cardiovascular disease [103, 229–232]

Syndrome/disease	Usual CVS association	Non CVS findings
Alagille (arteriohepatic dysplasia)	PS	Prominent forehead, deep set eyes, vertebral anomalies, biliary hypoplasia
Anotia and facial palsy	VSD, PS	
Apert	VSD	Craniosynostosis, midfacial hypoplasia syndactyly
CHARGE	Tetralogy of Fallot	Colobomas heart defects, atresia of choana, retarded growth, genital hypoplasia, ear abnormalities, and/or hearing loss
Cockayne	Accelerated atherosclerosis	Retinal pigmentary abnormalities, dwarfism, photosensitivity, dermatitis
Cornelia de Lange	VSD, PDA	Micromelia, low set ears, synophrys, low IQ
Cri du Chat (short arm deletion 5)	VSD	Microcephaly, antimongiloid slant, a cat cry, mental retardation
Crouzon	PDA, coarctation aorta	Craniosynostosis, maxillary hypoplasia, ptosis with shallow orbits
Di George	Interrupted aortic arch, TOF, truncus arteriosus	Thymic and parathyroidic hypoplasia, abnormal facies
Ellis–van Creveld* (chondro-ectodermal dysplasia)	AV canal	Dwarfism, polydactyly dysplastic fingernails, poor dentition, knock knees
Fabry disease*	IHD, hypertrophic cardiomyopathy, CVA	Angiokeratomas of bathing trunk area including scrotum and penis, neuropathy
Hurler (gargolysm)	Mitral valve disease, IHD, cardiomyopathy	Corneal clouding, coarse facies, dwarfism, kyphosis, low IQ, 4th and 5th fingers curved inwards
Jaccoud's arthritis (chronic post-RF arthritis)	Mitral and/or aortic valve disease	MCP joints flexed; ulnar deviation and/or subluxation of 4th and 5th fingers, bony erosions of metacarpal heads [192]

(Continued)

(*Continued*)

Syndrome/disease	Usual CVS association	Non CVS findings
Kearnes–Sayre*	Heart block, cardiomyopathy	Ophthalmoplegia, ptosis, retinal pigmentation
Klinefelter (XXY)	ASD	Gynecomastia, hypogonadism, tall stature, long limbs
Klippel Feil	VSD	Cleft palate, torticollis, scoliosis, deafness, strabismus, hydrocephalus
Laurence–Moon—Biedl*	PDA, TGV	Retinal pigmentation, obesity, polydactyly, hypogonadism
Pierre Robin	Truncus arteriosus	Cleft palate, low set ears, hypoplastic mandible
Post Rubella	PDA, VSD	Congenital cataracts, microcephaly, deafness, physical and mental retardation
Riley–Day (familial dysautonomia)	Postural hypotension, recurrent hypertension	Sad expression on face, hypertelorism, defective lacrimation, slurred speech, scoliosis, pes cavus
Rubinstein–Taybi	PDA, PS	Broad thumbs and toes, hypoplastic maxilla, antimongiloid slant, large low set ears
Shprintzen (velocardiofacial)	VSD, TOF	Cleft palate, prominent nose, slender hands, learning disability
Trisomy 13*	VSD, dextroposition	Colobomas, low set ears, deafness, polydactyly, simian crease, cleft palate
Trisomy 18	VSD, PDA	Micrognathia low set ears, clenched fingers with index finger crossing over 3rd finger, feeble babies with a kitten like cry. Webbed neck
VATER	VSD	Vertebral anomalies, and atresia, tracheoesophageal fistula, radial, and renal anomalies

Abbreviations: ASD, atrial septal defect; IHD, ischemic heart disease; PDA, persistent ductus arteriosus; PS, pulmonic stenosis; RF, rheumatic fever; TGV, transposition of great vessels; TOF, tetralogy of Fallot. *Alluded to briefly in text.

Synopsis

Step 1: Detection of the physical signs

General observations

Is the patient excessively tall or short? Body build should be noted. Is the patient alert or somnolent? Are there any abnormalities in the gait? Note the clothing for evidence of weight change or tobacco use.

Head

Are there any facial features to suggest a collagen or endocrine disorder such as butterfly eruption or exophthalmos, respectively? A masklike face may suggest Parkinsonism, scleroderma, or myotonia dystrophica, whereas a vacant expression suggests Down syndrome.

Are the eyes widely spaced apart (hypertelorism)? Do the conjunctiva appear pale or brick red? Are there any xanthelasma, waxy eyelid plaques, or drooping eyelids? Is the sclera discolored (e.g., blue or yellow)? Is there an Argyll Robertson pupil or subluxation of the lens? Is there an arcus corneae (unilateral or bilateral)? Fundi should be checked for hypertension, diabetes, dyslipidemias, or embolic changes due to carotid artery disease or IE.

Is there unilateral temporal artery prominence to suggest ipsilateral carotid disease or temporal arteritis? Skin findings such as malar flush, angiofibromata, slate gray pigmentation due to amiodarone, lupus pernio, facial edema, or premature aging should be noted.

The mouth should be inspected for dental hygiene or enamel erosions, gum hyperplasia, widely spaced teeth, macroglossia, tongue angiomata, or sublingual cyanosis. Are there any tonsillar lesions to suggest Tangier disease? Are there any petechiae or perforations of the hard palate? Is the nose saddle shaped? Do the ears show evidence of gout, alkaptonuria, or a diagonal crease sign?

Neck

Is there any webbing of the neck? Is the thyroid enlarged? Are there any surgical scars to suggest carotid or thyroid operations? Is there unilateral or bilateral jugular venous distention? Plucked chicken skin appearance of the neck?

Chest

Are there any deformities of the thoracic cage such as kyphoscoliosis, straight back syndrome, pectus excavatum, shield chest, or bamboo spine? Are there any surgical scars (thoracotomy, pacemaker, IV access site, or vascular surgery)? Are the ribs or sternum still intact? Is there any venous collateral circulation on the chest wall to suggest SVC syndrome? Is there gynecomastia?

Upper extremity

The hand should be examined for

(a) *Size and shape*: Acromegaly (spade like), Marfan syndrome (arachnodactyly), rheumatoid arthritis with an ulnar drift, Ehlers–Danlos syndrome with hyperextensible joints, Holt–Oram syndrome with fingerized thumb. Absent digits or deformed digits are also noted. Is there clubbing?

(b) *Edema*: Superior vena cava syndrome, thoracic outlet syndrome.

(c) *Neuromuscular disease*: Myotonia dystrophica, fine tremor of hyperthyroidism.

(d) *Color change*: Tobacco tar staining, cyanosis of nail beds, Raynaud's phenomenon, Osler's nodes, Janeway lesions, tissue necrosis associated with vasculitis.

(e) *Nail abnormalities*: Splinter hemorrhages, Terry's nails, red lunula, onycholysis, subungal fibromas.

(f) *Palmar changes*: Palmar erythema, simian crease, yellow palmar creases.

(g) *Temperature change*: Warm hands (e.g., hyperthyroidism) cold hands (e.g., vasculitis, arterial occlusion).

Are there any xanthomas (elbows, hands), surgical scars (brachial artery cut down, radial artery harvesting site for CABG); venous tracks from IV drug abuse or AV fistula?

Abdomen

Is there ascites or central obesity? Is liver visibly enlarged? Is there prominent venous collateral circulation due to IVC obstruction? Any signs of red abdominal striae of Cushing's disease; flank, periumbilical, or rectus sheath ecchymoses; swimming trunk skin eruption of Fabry's disease?

Back

Deformities such as kyphoscoliosis or bamboo spine are noted. The skin lesions of neurofibromatosis or eruptive xanthoma are often seen here. Any radiation injuries cause a dermatitis, skin necrosis, or myopathy?

Lower extremities

Skin lesions of erythema marginatum (thighs), erythema nodosum (legs), keratoderma, blennorrhagica, or Janeway lesions (soles of feet) are noted. Are skin popping sites (legs, thighs) seen?

Is there leg swelling (unilateral or bilateral)? Does the leg swelling pit or is it firm? Note evidence of pseudohypertrophy of calf muscles and Saber shins. Xanthomas of the nodular or tendinous type should be noted. Check for evidence of vascular insufficiency and gangrene of toes.

Step 2: Correlate the physical signs associated with the bracketed cardiovascular entity

1 *Congenital heart disease*: Holt–Oram syndrome (atrial septal defect); Down syndrome (atrioventricular canal defect, ventricular septal defect, persistent ductus arteriosus); Turner syndrome (coarctation of the aorta); Central cyanosis, poly-cythemia, and clubbing point to a right-to-left shunt.

2 *Vascular disease*: Hypertension, hyperlipidemia, smoking, diabetes, and obesity are detectible as CAD risk factors. Coronary artery disease may also be suspected in the presence of an ear-crease sign, evidence of mediastinal radiation, progeria, polycythemia, PXE, Tangier disease, acromegaly, longstanding rheumatoid arthritis, SLE, and in a cocaine addict.

Obstructive sleep apnea, polyarteritis nodosa, von Recklinghausen's disease, Cushing's syndrome, acromegaly, and gout are associated with hypertension.

Arcus corneae, xanthoma, lipemia retinalis suggest hyperlipidemia. Hyperlipidemia is seen in acromegaly and myxedema. Olivarius's sign, unilateral arcus corneae, and a Hollenhorst plaque occur in internal carotid artery disease.

Marfan and Ehlers–Danlos syndromes are associated with aortic aneurysms/rupture. Obstructive sleep apnea, sarcoidosis, scleroderma, and tricuspid regurgitation are associated with pulmonary hypertension. The Shy–Drager syndrome gives rise to postural hypotension.

Limb ischemia/necrosis may be due to atherosclerosis, cholesterol embolism, Buerger's disease, diabetes, Raynaud's phenomenon, or a collagen disease.

Facial edema, neck vein distention, prominent venous collateral circulation on the chest wall, and venous stars are seen in the superior vena cava syndrome, whereas prominent abdominal venous collateral circulation, leg edema, and possibly ascites point to the inferior vena cava syndrome.

Patients with the Osler–Weber–Rendu syndrome may have a pulmonary AV fistula.

3 *Infective endocarditis*: The physical signs are Roth spots, retinal hemorrhages, subungal hemorrhages, petechiae involving the conjunctiva or palate, Osler's nodes, and Janeway lesions. There may be valvular regurgitation (aortic, mitral, or tricuspid).

4 *Valvular heart disease*: Carcinoid syndrome, pulmonary hypertension (tricuspid regurgitation); Carcinoid, LEOPARD, and Noonan's syndromes (pulmonic stenosis); Osteogenesis imperfecta, PXE, Marfan syndrome, and IE (mitral regurgitation); PXE, Ehlers–Danlos syndrome, and Marfan syndrome (mitral valve prolapse syndrome); Marfan, Reiter's, ankylosing spondylitis, tertiary syphilis, IE, and osteogenesis imperfecta (aortic regurgitation); Ochronosis and Paget's disease of bone (aortic stenosis); LEOPARD syndrome (hypertrophic cardiomyopathy); William's syndrome (supravalvular aortic stenosis).

5 *Heart failure*: Patients with heart failure may have peripheral cyanosis, edema, elevated jugular venous pressure, leuconychia, and mild jaundice (hypertension, CAD, valvular heart disease, myocarditis, myocardiopathy, or pericardial disease may be the underlying cause of heart failure). High output failure occurs in Paget's disease, hyperthyroidism, beriberi, anemia, and AV fistula.

6 *Myocardial and pericardial disease*: Hemochromatosis, muscular dystrophy, Friedreich's ataxia, hyperthyroidism, amyloidosis, ankylosing spondylitis (cardiomyopathy); Rheumatic fever, Reiter's syndrome (myocarditis); Scleroderma, dermatomyositis, and sarcoidosis (pericarditis); Myxedema (pericardial effusion and possibly tamponade).

7 *Heart block*: Sarcoidosis, gout, rheumatic fever, Reiter's syndrome, SLE, and ankylosing spondylitis may be associated with atrioventricular block.

8 *Cardiac tumors*: Cardiac tumors may occur in neurofibromatosis, tuberous sclerosis, and LAMB syndrome.

References

1 Fitzgerald FT. Physical diagnosis skills: clues from the patient's appearance and belongings. *Consultant* 1996; **36**: 1539–1554.

2 Fitzgerald FT, Tierney LM, Jr. The bedside Sherlock Holmes. *West J Med* 1982; **137**: 169–175.

3 Steinberg I. A simple screening test for the Marfan syndrome. *Am J Roentgen* 1966; **97**: 118–124.

4 Walker BA, Murdoch JL. The wrist sign. A useful physical finding in the Marfan syndrome. *Arch Intern Med* 1970; **126**: 276–277.

5 Pyeritz RE, Gasner C. *The Marfan Syndrome*, 4th edn. National Marfan Foundation, New York, 1994.

6 Pyeritz RE. The Marfan syndrome. *Ann Rev Med* 2000; **51**: 481–510.

7 Rudolph AM, Hoffman JIE, Rudolph CD. *Rudolph's Pediatrics*, 20th edn. Appleton & Lange, Stamford, CT, 1996: 1782.

8 White NJ, Winearls CG, Smith R. Cardiovascular abnormalities in osteogenesis imperfecta. *Am Heart J* 1983; **106**: 1416–1420.

9 Wong RS, Follis FM. Shively BK *et al*. Osteogenesis imperfecta and cardiovascular diseases. *Ann Thorac Surg* 1995; **60**: 1439–1443.

10 Bailey H. *Demonstration of Physical Signs in Clinical Surgery*, 13th edn. John Wright & Sons Ltd., Bristol, 1960: 802.

11 Hultgen HN. Osteitis deformans (Paget's disease) and calcific disease of the heart valves. *Am J Cardiol* 1998; **81**: 1461–1464.

12 Arnalich F, Plaza JA, Sobrino J *et al*. Cardiac size and function in Paget's disease of bone. *Int J Cardiol* 1984; **5**: 491–505.

13 Fraser RS, Colman N, Muller NL, Pare' PD. Obesity hypoventilation syndrome. In: *Fraser & Pare's Diagnosis of Diseases of the Chest*, 4th edn. W.B. Saunders, Philadelphia, 1999: 3053.

14 Victor M, Ropper AH. *Adams & Victor's Principles of Neurology*, 7th edn. McGraw Hill, New York, 2001: 1145.

15 Mandell GL, Bennett JE, Dolin R. Syphilis. In: *Mandell, Douglas & Bennett's Principles & Practice of Infectious Diseases*, 4th edn. Churchill Livingstone, New York, 1995: 2125.

16 Cuetter AC, Pearl W, Ferrans VJ. Neurological conditions affecting the cardiovascular system. *Curr Probl Cardiol* 1990; **15**: 475–568.

17 Soffer A. Smokers faces. Who are the smokers? *Arch Intern Med* 1986; **146**: 1496.

18 Daniell MW. Smoker's wrinkles: a study in the epidemiology of crow's feet. *Ann Intern Med* 1971; **75**: 873–880.

19 Allander E, Bjornsson OJ, Kolbeinsson A *et al*. Incidence of xanthelasma in the general population. *Int J Epidemiol* 1972; **1**: 211.

20 Nardone DA, Roth KM, Mazur DJ *et al*. Usefulness of physical examination in detecting the presence or absence of anemia. *Arch Intern Med* 1990; **150**: 201–204.

21 Turner RWD. General observation of the patient. In: Friedberg CK (ed.), *Physical Diagnosis in CVS Disease*. Grune & Stratton, New York, 1969: 1–15.

22 Scheld WM, Sande MA. Endocarditis and intravascular infections. In: Mandell GL, Bennett JE, Dolin R (eds.), *Principles & Practice of Infectious Diseases*, 4th edn., Part 2. Churchill Livingstone, New York, 1995: 748.

23 Chan CC, Green WR, de la Cruz ZC *et al*. Ocular findings in osteogenesis imperfecta congenita. *Arch Ophthalmol* 1982; **100**: 1459–1463.

24 Roy FM. Blue sclera. In: *Ocular Differential Diagnosis*, 3rd edn. Lea & Febiger, Philadelphia, 1984: 277.

25 Barchiesi BJ, Eckel RH, Ellis PP. The cornea and disorders of lipid metabolism. *Surv Ophthalmol* 1991; **36**: 1–22.

26 Smith JL, Susac JO. Unilateral arcus senilis: sign of occlusive disease of the carotid artery. *JAMA* 1973; **226**: 676.

27 Roy FH. Hypertelorism. In: *Ocular Differential Diagnosis*, 3rd edn. Lea & Febiger, Philadelphia, 1984: 18–21.

28 Cross HE, Jensen AD. Ocular manifestations in the Marfan syndrome and homocystinuria. *Am J Ophthalmol* 1973; **75**: 405–420.

29 Bostom AG, Selhub J. Homocysteine and arteriosclerosis. Subclinical and clinical disease associations. *Circulation* 1999; **99**: 2361–2363.

30 Sapira JD. An internist looks at the fundus oculi. *Dis Mon* November 1984; **30**: 1–64.

31 Kanski JJ. *Clinical Ophthalmology*, 4th edn. Butterworth, Oxford, 1999: 495–497.

32 Wong TY, Mitchell P. Current concepts: hypertensive retinopathy. *N Engl J Med* 2004; **351**: 2310–2317.

33 Bourke K, Patel MR, Prisant LM *et al.* Hypertensive choroidopathy. *J Clin Hypertens* 2004; **6**: 471–472.

34 Kaye D (ed.). *Infective Endocarditis*, 2nd edn. Raven Press, New York, 1992.

35 Blumenthal EZ, Zamir E. Roth's spots. *Circulation* 1999; **99**: 1271.

36 Fisher CM. Facial pulses in internal carotid artery occlusion. *Neurology* 1970; **20**: 476–478.

37 Hellman DB. Temporal Arteritis. A cough, toothache, and tongue infarction. *JAMA* 2002; **287**: 2996–3000.

38 Manolis AS, Varriale P, Ostrowski RM. Hypothyroid cardiac tamponade. *Arch Intern Med* 1987; **147**: 1167–1169.

39 McKenzie JM, Zakarija M. Hyperthyroidism. In: De Groot LJ (ed.), *Endocrinology*, 3rd edn. W.B. Saunders, Philadelphia, 1995: 676–712.

40 Thorner MO, Vance ML. Acromegaly. In: *William's Textbook of Endocrinology*, 9th edn. W.B. Saunders, Philadelphia, 1998: 298–299.

41 David DS, Grieco MH, Cushman P. Adrenal glucocorticoids after 20 years. A review of their clinically relevant consequences. *J Chronic Dis* 1970; **22**: 637–711.

42 Plotz PH. Moderator. Current concepts in the idiopathic inflammatory myopathies: polymyositis, dermatomyositis and related disorders. *Ann Intern Med* 1989; **111**: 143–157.

43 Katayama I, Sawada Y, Nishioka K. Facial fold erythema—dermatomyositis: seborrheic pattern of dermatomyositis. *Br J Dermatol* 1999; **140**: 978–979.

44 Mandell BF, Hoffman GS. Dermatomyositis. In: *Braunwald's Heart Disease*, 7th edn. W.B. Saunders, Philadelphia, 2005:2114.

45 Follansbee WP. The cardiovascular manifestation of systemic sclerosis (scleroderma). *Curr Probl Cardiol* May 1986; **11**: 245–298.

46 Anuari A, Graninger W, Schneider B *et al.* Cardiac involvement in systemic sclerosis. *Arthritis Rheum* 1992; **35**: 1356–1361.

47 Fitzpatrick TB, Johnson RA, Wolff K *et al.* DLE. In: *Color Atlas and Synopsis of Clinical Dermatology*, 4th edn. McGraw Hill, New York, 2001: 361–367.

48 Moder KE, Miller TD, Tazelaar HD. Cardiac involvement in systemic lupus erythematosus. *Mayo Clin Proc* 1999; **74**: 275–284.

49 Doherty NE, Siegel RJ. Cardiovascular manifestations of systemic lupus erythematosus. *Am Heart J* 1985; **110**: 1257–1265.

50 Roberts WC, High ST. The heart in systemic lupus erythematosus. *Curr Probl Cardiol* 1999; **24**: 1–56.

51 Karrar A, Sequeria W, Block JA. Coronary artery disease in systemic lupus erythematosus: a review of the literature. *Semin Arthritis Rheum* 2001; **30**: 436–443.

52 Dhond MR, Matayoshi A, Laslett L. Coronary artery aneurysms associated with systemic lupus. *Clin Cardiol* 1999; **22**: 373.

53 Solinger AM. Drug related lupus. Clinical and etiological considerations. *Rheum Dis Clin North Am* 1988; **14**: 187–202.

54 Hardman JG, Limbird LE, Molinoff PB, Ruddon RW, Gilman AG. *Goodman & Gillman's the Pharmacological Basis of Therapeutics*, 9th edn. McGraw-Hill, New York, 1996: 868.

55 Rudolph AM, Hoffman JIE, Rudolph CD. Down syndrome. In: *Rudolph's Pediatrics*, 20th edn. Appleton & Large, Stamford, CT, 1996: 298.

56 Tandon R, Edward JE. Cardiac malformation associated with Down syndrome. *Circulation* 1973; **47**: 1349–1355.

57 Grumbach MM, Conte FA. Noonan's syndrome. *William's Textbook of Endocrinology*, 9th edn. W.B. Saunders, Philadelphia, 1998: 1355.

58 Burch M, Sharland M, Shinebourne E *et al.* Cardiologic abnormalities in Noonan syndrome. Phenotypic diagnosis and echocardiographic assessment of 118 patients. *J Am Coll Cardiol* 1993; **22**: 1189–1192.

59 Purvis-Smith SG. The Sydney line: a significant sign in Down's syndrome. *Aust Paediatr J* 1972; **8**: 198–200.

60 Gorlin RJ, Anderson RC, Blaw M. Multiple lentigenes syndrome. *Am J Dis Child* 1969; **117**: 652–662.

61 Woywodt A, Welzel J, Haase H *et al.* Cardiomyopathic Lentiginosis/LEOPARD syndrome presenting as sudden cardiac arrest. *Chest* 1998; **113**: 1415–1417.

62 Perloff JK. The heart in neuromuscular disease. *Curr Probl Cardiol* 1986; **11**: 511–557.

63 Leung DYM, Meissner HC. The many faces of Kawasaki syndrome. *Hosp Pract* January 2000; **35**: 77–94.

64 Doi YL, Furuno T, Takata J *et al.* Late consequences of Kawasaki disease. Images in cardiovascular medicine. *Circulation* 1996; **94**: 231–232.

65 Hijazi ZM, Udelson JE, Snapper H *et al.* Physiological significance of chronic coronary aneurysms in patients with Kawasaki disease. *J Am Coll Cardiol* 1994; **24**: 1633–1638.

66 Onouchi Z, Shimazu S, Kiyosawa N *et al.* Aneurysms of the coronary arteries in Kawasaki disease. An angiographic study of 30 cases. *Circulation* 1982; **66**: 6–13.

67 Weiner DM, Ewalt DH, Roach ES *et al.* Tuberous sclerosis complex: a comprehensive review. *J Am Coll Surg* 1998; **187**: 548–561.

68 Smith MC, Watson GH, Patel RG *et al.* Cardiac rhabdomyomata in tuberous sclerosis: their course and diagnostic value. *Arch Dis Child* 1989; **64**: 196–200.

69 Kwiatkowski DJ, Short P. Tuberous sclerosis. *Arch Dermatol* 1994; **130**: 348–354.

70 Gomez MR (ed.). *Tuberous Sclerosis*. Raven Press, New York, 1988: 147–158.

71 Rhodes AR, Silverman RA, Harrist TJ *et al.* Mucocutaneous lentigines, cardiomucocutaneous myxomas, and multiple blue nevi: the Lamb syndrome. *J Am Acad Dermatol* 1984; **10**: 72–82.

72 Vidaillet HJ, Jr, Seward JB, Fyke FE *et al.* "Syndrome Myxoma": a subset of patients with cardiac myxoma associated with pigmented skin lesions and peripheral and endocrine neoplasms. *Br Heart J* 1987; **57**: 247–255.

73 Casey M, Mah C, Merliss AD *et al.* Identification of a novel genetic locus for familial cardiac myxomas and Carney complex. *Circulation* 1998; **98**: 2560–2566.

74 George WM. Cutaneous findings related to cardiovascular disorders. *Int J Dermatol* 1998; **37**: 161–172.

75 Marinella MA. Red scalp sign [letter]. *Mayo Clin Proc* 2003; **78**: 252.

76 Saif MW, Khan U, Greenberg BR. Cardiovascular manifestations of myeloproliferative disorders: a review of the literature. *Hosp Physician* July 1999: 43–54.

77 Grant P, Patel P, Singh S. Acute myocardial infarction secondary to polycythemia in a case of cyanotic congenital heart disease. *Int J Cardiol* 1985; **9**: 108–110.

78 Rubinov A, Cohen AS. Skin involvement in generalized amyloidosis. *Ann Intern Med* 1978; **88**: 781–785.

79 Braverman IM. Amyloidosis. In: *Skin Signs of Systemic Disease*, 3rd edn. W.B. Saunders, Philadelphia, 1998: 190–197.

80 Gertz MA, Lacy MQ, Dispenzieri A. Amyloidosis: recognition, confirmation, prognosis and therapy. *Mayo Clin Proc* 1999; **74**: 490–494.

81 Strickman NE, Rossi PA, Massumkhani GA *et al.* Carcinoid heart disease: a clinical pathologic and therapeutic update. *Curr Probl Cardiol* 1982; **6**: 4–42.

82 Wood P. An appreciation of mitral stenosis. *Br Med J* 1954; **1**: 1051–1063 and 1113–1124.

83 Ricca J. Obstruction of the superior vena caval system: an extensive review. *N Y State J Med* 1959; **59**: 4171–4177.

84 Parish JM, Marschlke RF, Dines DE *et al.* Etiologic considerations in superior vena cava syndrome. *Mayo Clin Proc* 1981; **56**: 407–413.

85 Blackburn T, Dunn M. Pacemaker-induced superior vena cava syndrome: consideration of management. *Am Heart J* 1988; **116**: 893–896.

86 Wallace C, Siminoski K. The Pemberton sign. *Ann Intern Med* 1996; **125**: 568–569.

87 Norcross CQ, Auwaerter PG. The Pemberton and Maroni signs [letters]. *Ann Intern Med* 1997; **126**: 915–916.

88 Kaplan AP, Greaves MW. Angioedema. *J Am Acad Dermatol* 2005; **53**: 373–388.

89 Silverman ME. Supravalvular aortic stenosis (William's syndrome). *Cardiovasc Med* 1985; **10**: 57–61.

90 Zalzstein E, Moes CAF, Musew NN *et al.* Spectrum of cardiovascular anomalies in Williams–Beuren syndrome. *Pediatr Cardiol* 1991; **12**: 219–223.

91 Harris L, McKenna WJ, Rowland E *et al.* Side effects of long-term Amiodarone therapy. *Circulation* 1983; **67**: 45–51.

92 Blackshear JL, Randle HW. Reversibility of blue-gray cutaneous discoloration from amiodarone. *Mayo Clin Proc* 1991; **66**: 721–726.

93 Sra J, Bremner S. Amiodarone skin toxicity. Images in cardiovascular medicine. *Circulation* 1998; **97**: 1105.

94 James DG, Neville E, Siltzbach LE *et al.* A worldwide review of sarcoidosis. *Ann N Y Acad Sci* 1976; **278**: 321–334.

95 Matsui Y, Iwai K, Tachibana T *et al.* Clinical pathological study of fatal myocardial sarcoidosis. *Ann N Y Acad Sci* 1976; **278**: 455–469.

96 Roberts WC, McAllister HA, Ferrans VJ. Sarcoidosis of heart. *Am J Med* 1977; **63**: 86–108.

97 Steere AC, Bartenhagen NH, Craft JE. The early clinical manifestations of Lyme disease. *Ann Intern Med* 1980; **93**: 76–82.

98 Steere AC, Batsford WP, Weinberg M *et al.* Lyme carditis. Cardiac abnormalities of Lyme disease. *Ann Intern Med* 1980; **93**: 8–16.

99 Frank ST. Aural sign of coronary artery disease. *N Engl J Med* 1973; **289**: 327–328.

100 Eber B, Delgado P. More on the diagonal earlobe crease as a marker of coronary artery disease. *Am J Cardiol* 1993; **72**: 861.

101 Wagner RF, Reinfold HB, Wagner KD *et al.* Ear-canal hair and the ear-lobe crease as predictors for coronary artery disease. *N Engl J Med* 1984; **311**: 1317–1318.

102 Messerli FH, Frohlich ED, Dreslinski GL *et al.* Serum uric acid in essential hypertension. *Ann Intern Med* 1980; **93**: 817–821.

103 Sternberg MA, Neufeld HN. Physical diagnosis in syndromes with cardiovascular disease. In: Friedberg CK (ed.), *Physical Diagnosis in CVS Disease.* Grune & Stratton, New York, 1969: 16–40.

104 Fuster V, Alexander RW, O'Rourke RA (eds.). Low slung ears. In: *Hurst's the Heart*, 10th edn. McGraw-Hill, New York, 2001: 205.

105 Kenny D, Ptacin M, Bamrah VS *et al.* Cardiovascular ochronosis: a case report and review of the medical literature. *Cardiology* 1990; **77**: 477–483.

106 Blount SG, Jr. Cyanosis: pathophysiology and differential diagnosis. In: Friedberg CK (ed.), *Pathophysiology and Differential Diagnosis in Cardiovascular Disease.* Grune & Stratton, New York, 1971: 89–99.

107 Peery WH. Clinical spectrum of hereditary hemorrhagic telangiectasia (Osler–Weber–Rendu disease). *Am J Med* 1987; **82**: 989–997.

108 Swanson KL, Prakash UBS, Stanson AW. Pulmonary arteriovenous fistulas: Mayo Clinic Experience. *Mayo Clin Proc* 1999; **74**: 671–680.

109 Kurnick PB, Heymann WR. Coronary artery ectasia associated with hereditary hemorrhagic telangiectasia. *Arch Intern Med* 1989; **149**: 2357–2359.

110 Bouchier IAD, Ellis H, Fleming PR. Acute and chronic swelling of tongue. In: *French's Index of Differential Diagnosis*, 13th edn. Butterworth-Heinemann, London, 1996: 673.

111 Lapostolle F, Borron SW, Bekka R *et al.* Lingual angioedema after perindopril use. *Am J Cardiol* 1998; **81**: 523.

112 Wagner WO. Angioedema: frightening and frustrating. *Cleve Clin J Med* 1999; **66**: 203–205.

113 Sabroe RA, Kobza Black A. Angiotensin-converting enzyme (ACE) inhibitors and angio-edema. *Br J Dermatol* 1997; **136**: 153–158.

114 Kostis JB, Kim HJ, Rysnak J *et al.* Incidence and characteristics of angioedema associated with enalapril. *Arch Intern Med* 2005; **165**: 1637–1642.

115 Meraw SJ, Sheridan PJ. Medically induced gingival hyperplasia. *Mayo Clin Proc* 1998; **73**: 1196–1199.

116 Steele RM, Schuna AA, Schreiler RT. Calcium antagonist-induced gingival hyperplasia. *Ann Intern Med* 1994; **120**: 663–664.

117 Mitchell-Lewis DA, Phelan JA, Kelly RB *et al.* Identifying oral lesions associated with crack cocaine use. *J Am Dent Assoc* 1994; **125**: 1104–1108.

118 Bains MK, Hosseini-Ardeholic M. Palatal perforations: past and present. 2 case reports and a literature review. *Br Dent J* 2005; **199**: 267–269.

119 Driscoll SE. A pattern of erosive carious lesions from cocaine use. *J Mass Dent Soc* 2003; **52**:12–14.

120 Parry J, Porter S, Scully C *et al.* Mucosal lesions due to oral cocaine use. *Br Dent J* 1996; **180**: 462–464.

121 Krutchkoff DJ, Eisenberg E, O'Brien JE *et al.* Cocaine-induced dental erosions [letter]. *N Engl J Med* 1990; **322**: 408.

122 Warner E. Cocaine abuse. *Ann Intern Med* 1993; **119**: 226–235.

123 Pitts WR, Lange RA, Cigarroa JE *et al.* Cocaine-induced myocardial ischemia and infarction: pathophysiology, recognition and management. *Prog Cardiovasc Dis* 1997; **40**: 65–76.

124 Andrews FFH. Dental erosion due to anorexia nervosa with bulimia. *Br Dent J* 1982; **152**: 89–90.

125 Hay WW, Hayward AR, Levin MJ *et al.* High-arched palate. In: *Current Pediatric Diagnosis and Treatment*, 14th edn. Appleton & Lange, Stamford, CT, 1999: 417.

126 Fredrickson DS, Altrocchi PH. Tangier disease. In: Aronson SM, Volk BW (eds.), *Cerebral Sphingolipidoses*. Academic Press, New York, 1962: 343–357.

127 Mahley RW, Weisgraber KH, Farese RV, Jr. Disorders of lipid metabolism. In: *William's Textbook of Endocrinology*, 9th edn. W.B. Saunders, Philadelphia, 1998:1134.

128 Komuro R, Yamashita S, Sumitsuji S *et al.* Tangier disease with continuous massive and longitudinal diffuse calcification in the coronary arteries. *Circulation* 2000; **101**: 2446–2448.

129 Pietrini V, Ruzzuto N, Vergani C. Neuropathy in Tangier disease: a clinicopathologic study and a review of the literature. *Acta Neurol Scand* 1985; **72**: 495–505.

130 Ranganathan N, Sivaciyan V, Saksena F. Jugular venous pulse. In: *The Art and Science of Cardiac Physical Examination*. Humana Press, Totowa, NJ, 2006: 67–111.

131 Smith KS. The kinked innominate vein. *Br Heart J* 1960; **22**: 110–116.

132 Campbell EJM. Physical signs of diffuse airways obstruction and lung distension. *Thorax* 1969; **24**: 1–3.

133 Rudolph AM, Hoffman JIE, Rudolph CD. Webbing of neck. In: *Rudolph's Pediatrics*, 20th edn. Appleton & Lange, Stamford, CT, 1996: 1782.

134 Berdahl LD, Wenstrom KD, Hanson JW. Web neck anomaly and its association with congenital heart disease. *Am J Med Genet* 1995; **56**: 304–307.

135 Leipala JA, Kaitila I. Apparently new syndrome of short stature, lumbar malsegmentation and minor facial anomalies in two brothers. *Am J Med Genet* 1994; **52**: 103–107.

136 Spinner NB, Biegel JA, Sovinsky L *et al.* 46, XX, 15p+ documented as dup (17p) by fluorescence in situ hybridization. *Am J Med Genet* 1993; **46**: 95–97.

137 Matsunaga K, Kubo M, Tsuji S *et al.* A case of deletion of the short arm of chromosome 18 associated with chronic polymyositis. *Rinsho Shinkeigaku* 1993; **33**: 980–984.

138 Lurie IW, Gurevich DB, Binkert F *et al.* Trisomy 17p11-pter: unbalanced pericentric inversion, inv(17) (p11 q25) in two patients, unbalanced translocations t (4;17) (q27;p11) in a new born and t (4;17) (p16; p11.2) in a fetus. *Clin Dysmorphol* 1995; **4**: 25–32.

139 Bacino CA, Schreck R, Fischel-Ghodsian N *et al.* Clinical and molecular studies in full trisomy 22; further delineation of the phenotype and review of the literature. *Am J Med Genet* 1995; **56**: 359–365.

140 Franks AG, Jr. Cutaneous aspects of cardiopulmonary disease. In: Fitzpatrick TB, Eisen AZ, Wolff K, Austen KF (eds.), *Dermatology in General Medicine*, 3rd edn. McGraw Hill Book, New York, 1997: 1981.

141 Lebwohl M, Halperin J, Phelps RG. Brief report: occult pseudoxanthoma elasticum in patients with premature cardiovascular disease. *N Engl J Med* 1993; **329**: 1237–1239.

142 Berry TJ. *The Hand as a Mirror of Systemic Disease*. F.A. Davis, Philadelphia, 1963: 193–204.

143 Gonzalez-Juanatey C, Llorca J, Testa A *et al.* Increased prevalence of severe subclinical atherosclerotic findings in long-term treated rheumatoid arthritis patients

without clinically evident atherosclerotic disease. *Medicine* 2003; **82**: 407–413.

144 Solomon DH, Karlson EW, Rimm EB *et al.* Cardiovascular morbidity and mortality in women diagnosed with rheumatoid arthritis. *Circulation* 2003; **107**: 1303–1307.

145 Ross EA, Perloff JK, Danovitch GM *et al.* Renal function and urate metabolism in late survivors with cyanotic congenital heart disease. *Circulation* 1986; **73**: 396–400.

146 Cooley WC, Graham JM, Jr. Down syndrome—an update and review for the primary pediatrician. *Clin Pediatr* 1991; **30**: 233–253.

147 Marks ML, Whisler SL, Clericuzio C *et al.* A new form of long QT syndrome associated with syndactyly. *J Am Coll Cardiol* 1995; **25**: 59–64.

148 Basson CT, Solomon SD, Weissman B *et al.* The clinical and genetic spectrum of the Holt–Oram syndrome (heart–hand syndrome). *N Engl J Med* 1994; **330**: 885–891.

149 Holt M, Oram S. Familial heart disease with skeletal malformations. *Br Heart J* 1960; **22**: 236–242.

150 Bohm M. Holt–Oram syndrome. *Circulation* 1998; **98**: 2636–2637.

151 Brockhoff CJ, Kober H, Tsilimingas N *et al.* Holt–Oram syndrome. *Circulation* 1999; **99**: 1395–1396.

152 Satoda M, Pierpont MEM, Diaz GA *et al.* Char syndrome, an inherited disorder with patent ductus arteriosus, maps to chromosome 6p12–p21. *Circulation* 1999; **99**: 3036–3042.

153 Coury C. Hippocratic fingers and hypertrophic osteoarthropathy. A study of 350 cases. *Br J Dis Chest* 1960; **54**: 202–209.

154 Fischer DS, Singer DH, Feldman SM. Clubbing, a review with emphasis on hereditary acropathy. *Medicine* 1964; **43**: 459–479.

155 Goodwin JR. Diagnosis of left atrial myxoma. *Lancet* 1963; **1**: 464–467.

156 Hansen-Flaschen J, Nordberg J. Clubbing and hypertrophic osteoarthropathy. *Clin Chest Med* 1987; **8**: 287–298.

157 Dorney ER. Unilateral clubbing of the fingers due to absence of the aortic arch. *Am J Med* 1955; **18**: 150–154.

158 Lovibond JL. The diagnosis of clubbed fingers. *Lancet* 1938; **1**: 363–364.

159 Waring WW, Wilkinson RW, Wiebe RA *et al.* Quantitation of digital clubbing in children. Measurements of casts of the index finger. *Am Rev Respir Dis* 1971; **104**: 166–174.

160 Regan GM, Tagg B, Thomson ML. Subjective assessment and objective measurement of finger clubbing. *Lancet* 1967; **1**: 530–532.

161 Shamroth L. Personal experience. *S Afr Med J* 1976; **50**: 297–300.

162 Lovell RRH. Observation on the structure of clubbed fingers. *Clin Sci* 1950; **9**: 299–317.

163 Carroll DG, Jr. Curvature of the nails, clubbing of the fingers and hypertrophic pulmonary osteoarthropathy. *Trans Am Clin Climatol Assoc* 1971; **83**: 198–208.

164 Schneiderman H. Digital clubbing due to idiopathic pulmonary fibrosis. *Consultant* 1996; **36**: 1249–1256.

165 Farzaneh-Far A. Pseudoclubbing. *N Engl J Med* 2006; **354**: e14.

166 Byrne JJ. *The Hand: Its Anatomy and Diseases*. CC Thomas, Springfield, 1959: 76, 194–195.

167 Steinbrocker O. The shoulder–hand syndrome: present perspective. *Arch Phys Med Rehabil* 1968; **49**: 388–395.

168 Lin YT, Yeh L, Oka Y. Pathophysiology of general cyanosis. *N Y State J Med* 1977; **77**: 1393–1396.

169 Silverman ME, Hurst JW. The hand and the heart. *Am J Cardiol* 1968; **22**: 718–728.

170 de Takats G, Fowler EF. Raynaud's phenomenon. *JAMA* 1962; **179**: 1–8.

171 Stern ES. The aetiology and pathology of acrocyanosis. *Br J Dermatol Syph* 1937; **49**: 100–108.

172 Adams SL, Gore M. Diagnostician's digit. A repercussion of percussion. *JAMA* 1997; **277**: 1168.

173 Huggins RH, Schwartz RA, Janniger CK. Vitiligo. *Acta Dermatoven APA* 2005; **14**: 137–145.

174 Michaelson ED, Walsh RE. Osler's nodes—a complication of prolonged arterial cannulation. *N Engl J Med* 1970; **283**: 472–473.

175 Proudfit WL. Skin signs of infective endocarditis. *Am Heart J* 1983; **106**: 1451–1453.

176 Olin JW, Young JR, Graor RA *et al.* The changing clinical spectrum of thromboangiitis obliterans (Buerger's disease). *Circulation* 1990; **82**(Suppl IV): IV3–IV8.

177 Fitzpatrick TB, Johnson RA, Wolff K. Vasculitis. In: *Color Atlas and Synopsis of Clinical Dermatology*, 4th edn. McGraw Hill, New York, 2001: 373–377.

178 Doughty RN, Haydock DA, Wattie J *et al.* Systemic embolism from a large ascending aortic aneurysm. *Circulation* 1998; **97**: 1421–1422.

179 Holzberg M, Walker HK. Terry's nails: revised definition and new correlations. *Lancet* 1984; **1**: 896–899.

180 Terry RC. Red half moons in cardiac failure. *Lancet* 1954; **11**: 842–844.

181 Sheehy TW. Disease by nail. *Resid Staff Physician* 1990; **36**: 57–72.

182 Fitzpatrick TB, Johnson RA, Wolff K. Blue-gray nails. In: *Color Atlas and Synopsis of Clinical Dermatology*, 3rd edn. McGraw Hill, New York, 1997: 498–499.

183 Scher RK, Daniel CR, III. *Nails: Therapy, Diagnosis, Surgery*, 2nd edn. W.B. Saunders, Philadelphia, 1997: 202.

184 Friedberg IM, Vogel LN. Thyrotoxicosis—onycholysis. In: *Werner & Ingbar's The Thyroid*, 6th edn. JB Lippincott, Philadelphia, 1986: 732.

185 Sherlock S, Dooley J. Palmar erythema. In: *Diseases of the Liver and Biliary System*, 10th edn. Blackwell Science, London, 1996: 81.

186 Brewer MB, Zech LA, Gregg RE *et al*. Type III Hyperlipoproteinemia: diagnosis, molecular defects, pathology and treatment. *Ann Intern Med* 1983; **98**: 623–640.

187 Schneiderman H. Tuberous xanthomas and pancreatitis associated with combined hypercholesterolemia and hypertriglyceridemia. *Consultant* 1996; **36**: 1014–1018.

188 Gotto AM. Triglyceride: the forgotten risk factor. *Circulation* 1998; **97**: 1027–1028.

189 Pineo GF, Hull RD. Adverse effects of Coumadin anticoagulants. *Drug Saf* 1993; **9**: 263–271.

190 Hirsh J, Dalen JE, Deykin D *et al*. Heparin: mechanism of action, pharmacokinetics, dosing considerations monitoring, efficacy and safety. *Chest* 1992; **102**(Suppl): 337S–351S.

191 Ranganathan N, Sivaciyan V, Saksena F. Precordial pulsations. In: *The Art and Science of Cardiac Physical Examination*. Humana Press. Totowa, NJ, 2006: 113–139.

192 Fernandez-Herlihy L, Sopera B, Nadar A. Sternal hump (letters). *Mayo Clin Proc* 2004; **79**: 1590–1591.

193 Fred HL. Venous stars. *Hosp Pract* 1994; **29**: 14.

194 Pierce JA, Ebert RV. The barrel deformity of the chest, the senile lung and obstructive pulmonary emphysema. *Am J Med* 1958; **25**: 13–22.

195 Bates B, Bickley LS, Hoekelman RA. Thoracic cage shapes. In: *Physical Examination and History Taking*, 6th edn. JB Lippincott, Philadelphia, 1995: 253.

196 Shamberger RC. Congenital chest wall deformities. *Curr Probl Surg* 1996; **33**: 469–542.

197 Datey KK, Deshmukh MM, Engineer SD *et al*. Straight back syndrome. *Br Heart J* 1964; **26**: 614–619.

198 O'Neill TW. The heart in ankylosing spondylitis. *Ann Rheum Dis* 1992; **51**: 705–706.

199 Morris CA, Leonard CO, Dilts C *et al*. Adults with Williams syndrome. *Am J Med Genet* 1990; **6**(Suppl): 102–107.

200 Zacharias A, Habib RH. Delayed primary closure of deep sternal wound infections. *Tex Heart Inst J* 1996; **23**: 211–216.

201 Bouchier IAD, Ellis J, Fleming PR. Gynecomastia. In: *French's Index of Differential Diagnosis*, 13th edn. Butterworth-Heinemann, London, 1996: 249–250.

202 Karnes PS. Neurofibromatosis: a common neurocutaneous disorder. *Mayo Clin Proc* 1998; **73**: 1071–1076.

203 Alaeddini J, Frater RW, Shirani J. Cardiac involvement in neurofibromatosis. *Tex Heart Inst J* 2000; **27**: 218–219.

204 Zeihen, M. Spinal sign for heart disease. *Consultant* 2000; **40**: 1732.

205 Venance SL, Nicolle MW. Paraspinal atrophy in post-radiation lumbosacral radiculoplexopathy. *J Clin Neuromusc Dis* 2003; **5**: 49–50.

206 Om A, Ellahham S, Vetrovec GW. Radiation-induced coronary artery disease. *Am Heart J* 1992; **124**: 1598–1602.

207 Stewart JR, Fajardo LF, Gillette SM *et al*. Radiation injury to the heart. Special feature—Late effects. Consensus conference. *Int J Radiat Oncol Biol Phys* 1995; **31**: 1205–1211.

208 Heidenreich PA, Hancock SL, Lee BK *et al*. Asymptomatic cardiac disease following mediastinal irradiation. *J Am Coll Cardiol* 2003; **42**: 743–749.

209 Shope TB. Radiation-induced skin injuries from fluoroscopy. *Radiographics* 1996; **16**: 1195–1199.

210 Silen W. *Cope's Early Diagnosis of the Acute Abdomen*, 16th edn. Oxford University Press, Oxford, 1983: 119.

211 Cherry WB, Mueller PS. Rectus sheath hematoma. Review of 126 cases at a single institution. *Medicine* 2006; **85**: 105–110.

212 Desnick RJ, Brady R, Barranger J *et al*. Fabry disease, an under-recognized multisystemic disorder. Expert recommendations for diagnosis, management and enzyme replacement therapy. *Ann Intern Med* 2003; **138**: 338–346.

213 Fred HL. Obstruction of inferior vena cava. *Hosp Pract* September 1998; **33**: 43.

214 Runyon BA. Cardiac ascites. *J Clin Gastroenterol* 1988; **10**: 410–412.

215 Belch JJF, McCollum PT, Stonebridge PA *et al*. *Color Atlas of Peripheral Vascular Diseases*, 2nd edn. Mosby-Wolfe, London, 1996.

216 Anand SS, Wells PS, Hunt D *et al*. Does this patient have deep vein thrombosis? *JAMA* 1998; **279**: 1094–1099.

217 Doxiadis SA. Erythema nodosum in children. *Medicine* 1951; **30**: 283–334.

218 Sahn EE, Maize JC, Silver RM. Erythema Marginatum: an unusual histopathological manifestation. *J Am Acad Dermatol* 1989; **21**: 145–147.

219 Pettelot G, Bracco J, Barrillon D *et al*. Cholesterol embolization. Unrecognized complication of thrombolysis. *Circulation* 1998; **97**: 1522.

220 Blackshear JL, Jahanger A, Owenburg WA *et al*. Digital embolization from plaque-related thrombus in the thoracic aorta: identification with transesophageal echocardiography and resolution with warfarin therapy. *Mayo Clin Proc* 1993; **68**: 268–272.

221 Feder W, Auerbach RM. "Purple Toes": an uncommon sequela of oral Coumadin therapy. *Ann Intern Med* 1961; **55**: 911–917.

222 Schneiderman H. Atheromatous emboli and livedo. *Consultant* October 1992; **32**: 73–76.

223 Parker F. Xanthomas and hyperlipidemia. *J Am Acad Dermatol* 1985; **13**: 1–30.

224 Borrie P, Slack J. A clinical syndrome characteristic of primary Type IV-V hyperlipoproteinemia. *Br J Dermatol* 1974; **90**: 245–253.

225 Glueck CJ. Triglyceride analysis in hyperlipidemia. In: Rifkind BM, Levy RI (eds.), *Diagnosis & Therapy.* Grune & Stratton, New York, 1977: 22.

226 Polano MK. Xanthomatoses. In: Fitzpatrick TB, Eisen OZ, Wolff K *et al.* (eds.), *Dermatology in Medicine*, Vol 2, 4th edn. McGraw-Hill, New York, 1993: 1910.

227 Fitzpatrick TB, Johnson RA, Wolff K *et al.* Pretibial myxedema. In: *Color Atlas & Synopsis of Clinical Dermatology*, 4th edn. McGraw-Hill, New York, 2001: 421.

228 Weinberger HS, Ropes MW, Kulka JP *et al.* Reiters syndrome; clinical and pathological considerations. A long term study of 16 cases. *Medicine (Baltimore)* 1962; **41**: 35–91.

229 O'Rourke RA, Shaver JA, Silverman ME. Physical examination. In: Fuster V, Alexander RW, O'Rourke RA (eds.), *Hurst's The Heart*, 10th edn. McGraw Hill, New York, 2001: 203–218.

230 Friedman WF, Silverman N. Congenital heart disease in infancy and childhood. In: Braunwald E, Zipes DP, Libby P. *Heart Disease*, 6th edn. W.B. Saunders, Philadelphia, 2001: 1507–1508.

231 Brady RO, Schiffmann R. Clinical features of and recent advances in therapy for Fabry disease. *JAMA* 2000; **284**: 2771–2775.

232 Bywaters EGL. Relationship between heart and joint disease including "rheumatoid heart disease" and chronic post-rheumatic arthritis (type Jaccoud). *Br Heart J* 1950; **12**: 101–131.

General references

Chizner MA. *Classic Teachings in Clinical Cardiology*, Vol 1. A tribute to Proctor Harvey. Laennec Publishing, Cedar Grove, NJ, 1996.

Hurst JW. The examination of the heart: the importance of initial screening. *Dis Mon* May 1990; **36**(5): 245–313.

Perloff JK. *Physical Examination of the Heart and Circulation*, 3rd edn. W.B. Saunders, Philadelphia, 2000.

Ranganathan N, Sivaciyan V, Saksena F. *The Art and Science of Cardiac Physical Examination.* Humana Press, Totowa, NJ, 2006.

Index

Page numbers in italics refer to illustrations.